WORLD BANK DISCUSSION PAPER NO. 356

Evaluating Health Projects

Lessons from the Literature

Susan Stout
Alison Evans
Janet Nassim
Laura Raney
with substantial contributions from
Rudolpho Bulatao, Varun Gauri, and Timothy Johnston

The World Bank
Washington, D.C.

Discussion Papers present results of country analysis or research that are circulated to encourage discussion and comment within the development community. To present these results with the least possible delay, the typescript of this paper has not been prepared in accordance with the procedures appropriate to formal printed texts, and the World Bank accepts no responsibility for errors. Some sources cited in this paper may be informal documents that are not readily available.

Cover photography courtesy of Curt Carnemark and the World Bank.

ISSN: 0259-210X

Susan Stout is a senior evaluation officer and Alison Evans is an economist in the World Bank's Operations Evaluation Department. Janet Nassim is a population and reproductive health specialist in the Bank's Human Development Department. Laura Raney is a health economist in the Operations Evaluation Department.

Library of Congress Cataloging-in-Publication Data

Evaluating health projects : lessons from the literature / Susan Stout
 . . . [et al.].
     p.   cm.—(World Bank discussion papers ; 356)
   Includes bibliographical references.
   ISBN 0-8213-3881-1
   1. Public health—Evaluation.   2. Medical assistance—Evaluation.
3. Population assistance—Evaluation.   4. Nutrition policy—
Evaluation.   5. World Bank. Population, Health, and Nutrition
Dept.—Evaluation.   I. Stout, Susan, 1949–   . II. Series.
RA427.E93   1997

Contents

Annexes

Tables

Figures

Box

Foreword

From a modest start 25 years ago, the World Bank has become the world's largest lender in the health, nutrition, and population (HNP) sectors, and the Bank now plays a leading role as an advisor on national health policies, often advocating reforms to promote efficiency, cost-effectiveness, and responsiveness to emerging health problems. At the same time, the Bank is seeking ever greater evidence that its work produces results on the ground.

Morbidity, mortality, and fertility are determined by a complex array of factors in addition to health services. The most important are income, nutritional status, education, and the quality of the environment—particularly access to safe water and sanitation. The complexity of these relationships makes analysis of development effectiveness in the health sector particularly challenging. Data gaps further complicate the learning process.

This paper reviews lessons from the literature on approaches to the evaluation of health programs and policies. An important lesson of the review is that there are major gaps in our understanding of how to measure the effectiveness of health care systems. While progress has been made in the development of methods for the economic appraisal of investments in the sector, much has yet to be learned about how externally funded activities interact with the institutional and socioeconomic environment to improve health policies and outcomes.

Against this background, the paper describes how an assessment of the Bank's experience in the sector might be undertaken. The underlying thesis is that changes in health policy and improved health outcomes depend on the institutional incentives that drive health care system performance and on the demand for health services.

We hope that this paper will stimulate further work on development effectiveness in HNP by our development partners in donor and nongovernmental agencies, the research community, and borrowing country governments.

Robert Picciotto
Director General
Operations Evaluation

David de Ferranti
Director and Chair
Human Development Network

Abstract

The paper reviews the literature on the causes of observed changes in health and fertility levels, the evaluation of policies, and programs designed to accelerate these changes and presents the findings of earlier assessments of the Bank's work in subsectors of HNP. A framework delineating the relationships between Bank activities in the sector, the characteristics of the health care system, household behavior, and changes in health outcomes is presented, and four evaluative criteria for assessing the performance of health care systems are identified. Broadly, the approach anticipates that Bank activities are more successful, as measured by their influence on system performance, when they achieve an appropriate fit between the institutional incentives which determine the supply of health goods and services, the nature of those goods and services, and consumer demand. This paper ends with a description of a strategy for assessing the development effectiveness of the Bank's work in the health, population, and nutrition (HNP) sectors.

Abbreviations and Acronyms

BESD   Bank Economic and Social Database
CAS   Country Assistance Strategy
CBD   Community-based Distribution
CBR   Crude Birth Rate
CEM   Country Economic Memorandum
DALY   Disability-adjusted life-year
ESW   Economic Sector Work
FPPI   Family Planning Performance Index
ICB   International Competitive Banking
IEC   Information, education, and communication
IMR   Infant Mortality Rate
HNP   Health, Nutrition, and Population
MIS   Management Information System
NGO   Nongovernmental organization
OECD   Organization for Economic Cooperation and Development
OPS   Operational Policy Staff
PCR   Project Completion Report
PER   Public Expenditure Review
PHC   Primary Health Care
PPF   Project Preparation Facility
SAR   Staff Appraisal Report
STD   Sexually transmitted disease
SW   Staff Weeks
TFR   Total Fertility Rate
USAID   U.S. Agency for International Development
WHO   World Health Organization
WID   Women in Development

Acknowledgments

This paper was prepared by Susan Stout (OEDD1) with substantial contributions from Alison Evans (OEDD1), Laura Raney (OEDD1), Timothy Johnston (OEDD1), Varun Gauri (OEDD1), and Janet Nassim (HDD). Rudolpho Bulatao provided detailed advice and suggestions on the comparative framework detailed in Chapter 5 and the design of instruments to be used in the study. Roger Slade provided extensive comments and suggestions throughout the production of the paper. Philip Musgrove provided valuable comments on earlier drafts. External reviewers for this paper are: Dr. Henry Mosley, Professor of International Health, Johns Hopkins University; Dr. Jose-Luis Bobadilla, to whom this paper is dedicated and whose untimely death in October 1996 is a major loss to the international health field in general and to those working on the evaluation of effectiveness of donor interventions in the sector in particular, Senior Health Specialist, Inter-American Development Bank; Dr. Amy Tsui, Professor of Maternal and Child Health, School of Public Health, University of North Carolina at Chapel Hill and Director, the Evaluation Project; and Dr. N. Soekirman, former Deputy Director for Human Resources, BAPPENAS, Government of Indonesia. The paper also benefited from comments received and discussion during a review meeting held in the World Bank on September 17, 1996. Caroline McEuen edited the manuscript. Benjamin Crow provided administrative support.

1. Introduction and Overview

This paper outlines the background of the Bank's work in the health, nutrition, and population (HNP) sector and elaborates a strategy for the assessment of its effectiveness.[1] The Bank has been active in HNP since 1970; by the close of fiscal 1995, it had committed nearly US$10 billion to lending in the health sector and had initiated activities in eighty-nine countries. The pace of growth in the sector has accelerated significantly in the last six years, and it thus appears timely to launch an assessment of the effectiveness of these efforts.

As background to the presentation of a proposal of how best to approach such an assessment, which is presented in chapter 5, we will present an exploration of the literature on the causes of the changes that have been observed in health and fertility levels, the lessons learned from previous evaluations of policies and programs designed to accelerate these changes, and the findings of earlier assessments of the Bank's work in subsectors of HNP. The aim is to identify information that will be helpful in the identification of benchmarks of sectoral performance and effectiveness.

The next chapter presents a summary review of the trends in health and fertility and what is known about the causes of these changes. This serves as the basis for the proposed evaluation of policy and programs. Trends in mortality and fertility are, of course, determined by a complex interaction of deliberate programs as well as changes in income, education, and a range of other variables. Understanding the lessons of previous efforts to explain trends in mortality and fertility will provide a context for considering two questions: how much and what kind of health gains might occur because of changes exogenous to deliberate HNP policies? Also, are the gains achieved from any intervention more or less than they might have been in the absence of the programs?

The discussion begins with a brief recitation of the remarkable changes in both fertility and mortality during the last century; an effort is then made to consider the likely explanations for these changes—first in fertility, and second in mortality. Fertility and mortality are the major engines of overall population change. Falling death rates are generally followed—after a predictable lag—by changes in birth rates. The differences in the pace of change between these variables is a population's rate of natural increase. The chapter does not include the many different views of the social or economic consequences of ill health or high fertility beyond the recognition that mitigation of these consequences is the fundamental rationale for HNP policies and programs.

Changes in mortality and fertility are influenced by programs and policies, as well as by broader social and economic change. Determining how policy effects changes in these outcomes is the core evaluative problem in the HNP sector. Chapter 3 reviews the variety of approaches and methods that have been used to address this problem. The primary objective is to present an overview of the tools and methods that can be employed to evaluate population and health policies and to draw attention to the principle findings of this research. The purpose is to identify

---

1. The term health sector is used to include activities in each of the three major subsectors (health, nutrition, and population).

the kinds of evaluative tools that might be used to assess the development effectiveness of the Bank's HNP work.

The chapter begins with an overview of the evaluation tools and methods that have been used to assess the effectiveness of family planning programs, the primary instrument in population policy. A discussion of experiences in the evaluation of health programs follows the discussion of family planning program evaluation. The programs are dealt with in this order because fertility is a less complex variable, with fewer, and largely known, determinants, and because population policy concerns largely preceded the focus on health outcomes that is now prevalent in development policy.

In general, the chapter demonstrates that the literature on the evaluation of family planning programs is wider and more tractable than the information on health and disease control programs. Evaluation literature in the health field is dominated by studies of the effectiveness of specific interventions (for example, programs to improve the treatment of a particular disease, such as tuberculosis or AIDS) rather than evaluations of the performance of the sector as a whole. That mortality is the outcome of a large number of diseases and their preceding risk factors (particularly poor nutritional status) further complicates the health program evaluation literature. A further constraint on evaluation in the health sector derives from the paucity of reliable local estimates of health outcomes. Nevertheless, significant work has been completed in recent years to identify ways to overcome the difficulties inherent in using mortality data (when it is available) and to develop the necessary conceptual tools to enable the application of economic analysis in setting health priorities. These methods are also briefly introduced, although it is noted that these are of limited utility for ex post evaluation of the effectiveness of health programs.

A summary of the history of the Bank's involvement in the sector and the evolution of its principal policy recommendations are presented in chapter 4. Starting from an initial focus on population policy and the reduction of high fertility, the Bank's focus in the sector has broadened over the past twenty-five years to encompass the health sector as a whole. This evolution is reflected in a steadily growing portfolio of activities focused on an increasingly broad set of objectives. The paper summarizes the findings of a number of reviews of the Bank's HNP experiences and identifies principal lessons for the future.

Chapter 5 draws out the implications of the findings of chapters 2 through 4 and presents the design of a study that will help to answer the question of how to measure and assess the development effectiveness of the Bank's work in HNP. The chapter presents a framework delineating the relationships between Bank activities in the sector, the characteristics of the health care system, household behavior, and changes in health outcomes (morbidity, mortality, and fertility). Four evaluative criteria for assessing the performance of health care systems are identified: clinical/epidemiological effectiveness, accessibility and the distribution of services, consumer satisfaction, and economic efficiency. An approach to assessing the effectiveness of Bank activities relative to changes in the performance of health care systems, and to the degree possible changes in health outcomes, is presented.

2. Trends in Fertility and Mortality

Improved trends in mortality and fertility are, of course, the intended outcomes of population and health policies and programs. Yet, these trends beyond the policies and programs are determined by a complex interaction of changes in income, education, and a range of other variables. Understanding the lessons of previous efforts to explain trends in mortality and fertility provides a context for considering two questions. First, how much and what kind of health gains might occur because of changes exogenous to deliberate HNP nutrition policies? Second, are the gains achieved from any intervention more or less than they might have been in the absence of the programs?

Remarkable changes in both fertility and mortality have taken place during the past century. Falling death rates are generally followed, after a lag, by changes in birth rates—the difference the pace of change between these variables is the rate of natural increase. Mortality and fertility are interrelated. High fertility has implications for mortality because it is associated with closer spacing of children and greater risks of child and maternal mortality. High infant mortality is connected to demand for larger families to replace lost children. These linkages are examined in depth in a broad array of literature (Caldwell and others 1990; Bongaarts 1994).

Fertility

The past 200 years have witnessed the most remarkable change in human demographic patterns yet recorded—a shift from high, relatively uncontrolled fertility to low, controlled fertility throughout large parts of the world. The fertility transition started in Europe in the early nineteenth century and was followed in countries of European settlement in the second half of the century. The transition in fertility spread rapidly, particularly following the invention and diffusion of modern contraceptive technology in the 1960s. The transition is largely completed in most of East Asia, well under way in Southeast Asia, and is proceeding, although more slowly, in South and West Asia. Fertility in parts of India (Kerala, areas in Tamil Nadu) and Sri Lanka is at remarkably low levels. Although slower to start, the Middle East now has a downward trend in fertility; more recently, fertility began to diminish in Sub-Saharan Africa. Overall, the total fertility rate (TFR) in developing countries has fallen from 6.1 to 3.9 births for each woman since 1960. Fertility levels are lowest in East Asia (average about 2.4) and highest in Sub-Saharan Africa (6.6) (Ross and Frankenberg 1993). Contraceptive use has risen from about 10 percent to about 50 percent of all couples in the developing world (it averages about 70 percent in the Western industrial countries). There are major variations in fertility levels within countries as well.

Mortality

Mortality began to decline in Europe and North America about two centuries ago, although the descent was initially slow. In the United States, life expectancy in 1890 was approximately forty-nine years, and child mortality was about 180 for each 1,000 live births. Improvements accelerated significantly only in the first half of this century, and they have progressed more in the past forty years than in all of previous human history. In developing countries, life expectancy has increased from about forty to sixty-three years, and child mortality has fallen from about 280 to 106 for every 1,000 live births. Today, life expectancy in a high-income country is seventy-five years or more, while in Sub-Saharan Africa, where progress has been slowest, it is about fifty years (World Bank 1993) (see Table 2.1). As in fertility, declines in mortality have accelerated over the past thirty years. Data for developing countries show annual declines in child mortality of about 2 percent during the 1960s, about 3 percent during the 1970s, and more than 5 percent in the 1980s.

Table 2.1: Crude Death Rate and Life Expectancy at Birth, by Region, 1950–85

	Crude death rate (deaths per 1,000 persons annually)				Life expectancy at birth (years)	
	1950	1965	1980	1985–90	1950–55	1985–90
Sub-Saharan Africa	29.3	22.8	17.7	15.3	—	51.5
Middle East and North Africa	24.0	18.1	12.6	10.9	—	59.0
South Asia	28.8	20.6	14.5	12.2	38.9	55.8
East Asia (excluding China)	27.1	16.3	10.5	7.3		67.9
China	27.3	16.0	7.9	6.7	40.8	69.0
Latin America and the Caribbean	16.6	11.7	8.5	7.2		66.6
Developing countries					41.1	59.1
Industrial countries	10.5	9.6	9.1	9.3	65.8	73.1

— Not available.
Source: Birdsall 1995.

As in fertility, there are significant geographic and subregional differences in the levels and pace of change in mortality. Overall, China and other Asian countries have recorded the most rapid improvements, followed by the Middle East and Latin America. Sub-Saharan Africa has shown the least improvement, with a life expectancy that increased from about forty years in the early 1950s to about fifty-two today, although this pace is still faster than the rate of change experienced in parts of Europe in the nineteenth century. In both developing and high-income countries the bulk of the declines in mortality have been realized through the control of communicable diseases, particularly those of childhood, and the reduction of maternal and perinatal death.

Explaining Fertility and Health Transitions

Recent efforts to take stock of analytic progress (Caldwell 1990; Jamison and others 1993; World Bank 1993; Rashad and others 1995) provide a useful starting point for assembling observations about the nature and causes of transitions in fertility and health status. The findings presented here indicate areas of consensus among a wide range of theoretical and empirical studies.

Understanding Changes in Fertility

The most significant early attempt to explain trends in fertility was the construction of the so-called theory of the demographic transition. Briefly, this construction postulates that every society tends "to keep its vital processes in a state of balance such that population will replenish losses from death and grow to an extent deemed desirable by collective norms. These norms are flexible and readjust rather promptly to changes in the ability of the economy to support population" (Bogue 1969). Originally developed to explain the conditions that led to the significant acceleration in the pace of population growth that began in the 1930s, transition theory suggests that in societies where death rates are high, there is little need to regulate fertility, except to address the desires of individual couples, because high fertility is required to offset high mortality. In technologically advanced societies where death rates have been brought to a very low level, high birthrates come to be seen as dysfunctional, and the regulation of fertility and family size is increasingly identified as a collective good. Declines in fertility lag behind declines in mortality, resulting in a period of rapid population growth. The length of this period varies greatly among societies, depending on a combination of circumstances that will be unique in each case.

The strategies to predict fertility decline that emerged from this effort focused on two kinds of questions: classification of countries into groups according to the likely timing and pace of their demographic transition, and understanding the processes that translate declines in mortality into altered household behaviors, declines in desired family size, and, ultimately, the need or demand for family planning services. Work to address the first question led to a variety of schemes to identify the likelihood of a fertility decline in a given country and to anticipate the external finance and programmatic activity that would facilitate more rapid declines in fertility (see, for example, Berelson 1978).

Work to address the second question quickly overcame progress on the first with the introduction of the systematic application of household economic theory. The theory was systematically applied to achieve an understanding of the demand for children and work at both macroeconomic and microeconomic levels and to understand the influence of social and economic factors on fertility. At the macroeonomic level, the study of differential fertility patterns, based primarily on cross-sectional survey data, focuses on the relationship of educational attainment, particularly for girls, higher income, and urbanization with a decline in family size (see Cochrane 1979 for an early review of this literature). The Bank's 1984 *World Development Report* (*Population and Development*) provides a comprehensive assessment of this research.

At the microeconomic level, work by Bongaarts (1978) led to the development of a simple and validated model of the basic *proximate determinants* of fertility. The model demonstrates that four variables determine levels of fertility: age at marriage, duration of breastfeeding, use of contraception, and abortion. (It is worth noting that each of these variables has significant consequences for morbidity and mortality.) Socioeconomic and institutional variables affect fertility patterns through their influence on one or more of these determinants, as documented and elaborated through most of the subsequent research. As recently summarized by Gertler and Molyneaux (1994, p. 34):

> The most frequently observed fertility-reducing factors are those which apparently increase the cost of children by increasing the value of women's time (typically female "wages and education") and reducing contraceptive costs (prices and travel time to suppliers).

Two observations about this development are of interest. First, there is consensus within the field of fertility research on the validity of the proximate determinants model and, consequently, agreement that analyses of the effects of programmatic and policy measures on fertility need to specify how the action or activity translates into an influence on one or more of the proximate determinants. Although the relative importance of "development" and contraception as determinants is subject to continuing debate (see Gertler and Molyneaux 1994; Pritchett 1994; and Bongaarts 1995 for the latest elaborations of this issue), there is little question that any influence on fertility must operate through one of the four proximate determinants. This means that accurate modeling of the fertility transition is highly dependent on accurate historical data on both the levels and trends of socioeconomic change and the availability of family planning program inputs for the setting under study.

This leads to the second observation: efforts that adequately account for macroeconomic and microeconomic sources of variance in the evaluation of the impact of population policy and programs are few in number. Such studies have been possible only in the few national settings where sufficient time series of both socioeconomic and programmatic data are available.

Current Fertility Status

Despite the considerable progress that has been made in achieving fertility reductions throughout the developing world, high fertility continues to exert upward pressure on population growth rates in many countries. Excluding China, total fertility rates for the developing world, although lower than in 1960, are sufficiently high to double population growth in the next three decades (Bulatao 1993). More salient in today's policy environment, high fertility and sustained high levels of "unmet need" for contraception (measured as the proportion of couples who state a desire for no more children but are not actively using contraception), in combination with limited access to essential obstetric services, continue to pose threats to reproductive health. Although deliberate programs to increase access to contraception have significantly accelerated fertility decline in the past thirty years, much remains to be done. Fortunately, as detailed below, the considerable body of knowledge developed through evaluative studies of the performance of family planning programs offers several suggestions of how family planning programs can be made more effective and sustainable, even in resource-constrained environments.

Understanding Changes in Mortality and Health Status

Although there are few "easy" generalizations about the determinants of fertility change, there are even fewer about the determinants and future trends in mortality. In part, this is because fertility reflects a single, clearly defined biological event (birth), whereas death occurs through a multiplicity of socioeconomic and biological paths, making it difficult to meaningfully classify or measure "proximate" causes.[2] Nevertheless, three elements are clearly crucial to the transition in mortality: income growth, which allows people to buy more food, better housing, and more health care; improvements in medical technology, most notably the introduction of antibacterial drugs and new vaccines in the 1930s (and measles vaccine in the 1980s); and the introduction and diffusion of public health measures (particularly clean water, sanitation, and food regulation) and, especially important, *the diffusion of knowledge on the causes of poor health and what to do if a health-related problem develops*. In general, better-educated individuals and families with educated mothers experience significantly lower mortality than others. As in the case of fertility,

---

2. Mosley and Chen (1984), however, do attempt to define proximate determinants for mortality, concentrating on structural explanations, including improvements in maternal education, income, and urbanization.

efforts to improve education, particularly the education of girls, have major positive payoffs in the reduction of mortality.

Although change in income is a particularly strong structural correlate of mortality, the relationship between income growth and mortality decline is not monotonic. As summarized by Kunitz and Engerman (1992), several social and economic factors mitigate against a direct relationship between income and health, which makes it unrealistic to presume that "wealth will lead to health." Epidemiological factors, such as the association between prenatal and early childhood health status and adult mortality, create cohort effects that weaken the relationship between income and mortality. Sociological factors, including differences in attitudes and practices that affect women's status and education, work independently of income.

Several countries and subnational populations have experienced faster and more widespread declines in mortality than would be predicted by income alone. A series of papers sponsored by the Rockefeller Foundation (Halstead and others 1985) provide detailed documentation of experience in China; Costa Rica; Sri Lanka; and Kerala, India. In each of these cases, mortality has fallen radically below what might have been anticipated on the basis of changes in income. In-depth analysis of the factors that underlie these exceptional experiences suggests that social, political, and cultural factors contributed to the accelerated achievement of lower mortality in these low-income settings. Reviewing this set of sociopolitical experiences and the accompanying health service delivery systems, Caldwell (1986, p. 208) concludes:

> Unusually low mortality will be achieved if the following conditions hold: (1) sufficient female autonomy; (2) considerable inputs into *both* health services and education, both essentially of the modern or Western model, and with female schooling levels equaling or being close to male levels; (3) health services accessible to all no matter how remote, poor, or socially inferior to those providing them; (4) ensuring that the health services work efficiently, usually because of popular pressure (and, in addition, disciplining rural health workers by having a physician in charge); (5) providing either a nutritional floor or distributing food in some kind of egalitarian fashion; (6) achieving universal immunization; and (7) concentrating on the period before and after birth, usually by providing antenatal and postnatal health services and having deliveries performed by persons fully trained for this purpose, and often by health visitors calling on households so frequently that they not only provide advice and services but also play a decision making role in treatment.

The role of sociopolitical influences in enabling these populations to overcome the constraints of low income and limited "modernization" suggests that it is unlikely that any single "model PHC program" will fit the institutional and social environment of all settings. The consequences for public policy are significant, suggesting that progress in solving the health problems of the poor—including limited access to even the most basic health care and continuing threats from communicable disease—is significantly constrained by political influences on decisions regarding resource allocation, the structure of service delivery systems, and disease priorities. Building country-level capacity to define and evaluate possible approaches to achieve these "breakthrough conditions" may be a necessary first step to establishing more widespread progress in mortality decline.

The Epidemiological Transition and Future Trends

Recent research on mortality has been directed toward identifying patterns or mixes of causes of death across and within population groups and projecting probable future changes in the pattern of disease as an ingredient in anticipating health system needs and priorities. As summarized in background work for the 1993 *World Development Report*, health patterns, particularly those in the developing world, will be strongly influenced by recent and projected future declines in fertility and mortality as countries pass through the demographic transition (Jamison and others 1993). As fertility declines, the population ages, and the cause structure of death shifts to produce a transition in the nature and form of disease risks in what has become known as the *epidemiological transition.* Socioeconomic changes amplify the effects of population aging on patterns of risk. The shift from rural to urban living, for example, carries greater increased risks of injury related to motor vehicles, industrial accidents, and toxic chemicals. Chronic conditions such as cardiovascular diseases, cancer, and chronic obstructive pulmonary disease are also associated with increases in economic status and associated increases in the incidence of smoking, alcohol abuse, unhealthy diets, and sedentary lifestyles.

Because economic growth is neither steady nor even across population groups, the epidemiological transition does not occur evenly across a population. As a consequence, developing countries increasingly face *epidemiological polarization*—meaning that their health systems must develop the capacity to deal with the high incidence of communicable diseases, primarily among rural and poor groups, as well as significant increases in adult health problems and noncommunicable diseases among more urban and wealthier populations. The epidemiologic transition brings not only polarization, but also prompts an important shift in the burden of disease as the population continues to grow (based on built-in momentum, which maintains growth despite declines in fertility) and as noncommunicable diseases become dominant in the health profile of the country. The combination of these shifts requires corresponding shifts in the services delivered through the health care system. These changes in health technology can exert strong upward pressures on health care costs. In addition, as education improves, accessibility to information on health conditions increases, and the threshold at which health needs are translated into active demands on the health system is lowered, increasing the demand for health services (Jamison and others 1993).

Current Health Status in Developing Countries

Despite significant progress in recent decades, mortality risks remain high throughout the developing world. Table 2.2 summarizes recent data on the cause of death in industrial and developing countries in 1985 and as projected for 2015. Two points are noteworthy. First, the developing countries continue to face a significant burden of communicable disease and maternal and child health risks, which account for about 36 percent of all deaths, compared with about 9 percent in industrial countries. Second, current projections suggest that the burden of disease will shift toward a greater proportion of chronic and noncommunicable disease by the year 2015.

Table 2.2: Major Causes of Death in Industrial and Developing Countries, 1985 and 2015 (percent)

Cause of death	Industrial countries		Developing countries	
	1985	*2015*	*1985*	*2015*
Infections	9	7	36	19
Neoplasms	18	18	7	14
Circulatory problems	50	53	19	35
Pregnancy-related deaths	0	0	1	1
Perinatal problems	1	1	8	5
Injuries	6	5	8	7
Other	15	16	21	19
Total number of deaths (millions)	12.0	14.5	37.9	47.8

Source: Jamison and others (1993, p. 679).

Implications for Evaluation

Several of the findings of this review are relevant to development effectiveness in the HNP sector. First, it is clear that both socioeconomic change and deliberate policies and programs matter in determining outcomes. Paths to lower fertility and mortality vary among and between countries, but it is clear that levels and trends in female educational status, income, urbanization, and modern communication play a role in bringing about favorable shifts in population dynamics.

Second, although the fertility transition is under way throughout most of the developing world and is not likely to be reversed, high fertility continues to be an issue in many settings, particularly for health outcomes. Mortality is also declining, but changing age structures (another result of the fertility decline) and differential paces of socioeconomic development within and between countries contribute to a complex epidemiological mix. Many societies, particularly middle-income countries, now face the dual challenge of continuing to make progress against communicable diseases and dealing with persistent maternal and child health challenges, while also facing rapid growth in noncommunicable and chronic diseases that affect older and aging populations. These forces will exert growing pressures on already strained health budgets. Third, the shift in disease burden is not independent of income—the poor, and poor subgroups, experience the epidemiological transition more slowly than more well-off populations, largely because they are prey to poor information, limited access to educational opportunity, and limited basic health services.

Accordingly, assessments of performance in the HNP sector need to explicitly consider the context in assessing the outcome of a project or activity; particular attention must be given to the epidemiological and demographic status of each setting. Rather than seeking to generalize findings across all countries, or even across all projects in the portfolio, it is necessary to examine programmatic experience in a range of countries selected to represent varied positions along the epidemiological transition and the path of socioeconomic development.

Judgments on the relevance of particular investments must also focus on the distributional questions raised by inequities in health status. It is important not only to assess the degree of accuracy in identification of inequity in health status, but also to determine whether and how the resulting knowledge has shaped policy and project design.

3. Evaluating Programs to Influence Fertility and Health Outcomes

Changes in mortality and fertility are influenced by programs and policies, as well as by broader social and economic change. Determining how policy effects changes in these outcomes is the core evaluative problem in the HNP sector. This chapter provides an overview of the variety of approaches and methods that have been employed to address this problem. The primary objective is to present an overview of the tools and methods for evaluating population and health policies and to draw attention to the principal findings of this research.

The first task is to review the kinds of evaluative tools and methods that have been used to assess the effectiveness of family planning programs, the primary instrument in population policy. In general, the literature on the evaluation of family planning programs is wider and more tractable than the information available on health and disease control programs .There are two major reasons for this disparity: fertility is a less complex variable, with fewer and largely known determinants, and population policy concerns generally preceded the current focus on health outcomes in policy discussions of health sector priorities.

Next, attention turns to a discussion of the evaluation of health programs. In general, the evaluation literature in the health field is dominated by studies of the effectiveness of discrete interventions (for example, programs to improve the treatment of a particular disease, such as tuberculosis or AIDS) rather than of the performance of the sector as a whole. Mortality is an outcome of a large number of diseases and risk factors that are present before a morbid or disease condition, which creates grater complexity within the health program evaluation literature. A further constraint on evaluation in the health sector derives from the paucity of reliable local estimates of health outcomes. Nevertheless, significant work has been completed in recent years to identify ways to overcome the difficulties inherent in using mortality data (when it is available) and to develop the necessary conceptual tools to enable the application of economic analysis to the setting of health priorities. These methods are also briefly introduced, although it is noted that they are of limited utility for ex post evaluation of the effectiveness of health programs.

A concluding section of the chapter attempts to identify the major implications of the evaluation literature in defining and measuring the effectiveness of the Bank's HNP work, a topic that is treated in greater depth in chapter 5.

Measuring Family Planning Program Performance

The extensive literature evaluating family planning programs and chronicling the methods used dates from the initiation of the first large-scale national programs in the 1960s. For instance, the Taichung Experiment in Taiwan, China (Freedman and Takeshita 1969) used a true experimental design to assess the impact of family planning availability at the initiation of the Taiwan family planning program. Beyond establishing that family planning influenced contraceptive use in Taiwan, this study became a classic in the general impact evaluation literature and continues to be cited as an example of the application of experimental methods to social policy questions in developing countries. Many other forms of evaluation applicable to family planning have emerged in recent years. A compilation (Buckner and others 1995) of the large body of evaluation research in family planning classifies the many studies that have been completed into three major groups: process evaluations, the family planning performance index, and outcome evaluations.

Process Evaluation in Family Planning

Process evaluations of family planning programs focus on program implementation and the intermediate steps that determine how program inputs are transformed into outputs (contraceptive use) linked to the ultimate outcome of interest (decreased fertility). Two major kinds of methods have been used in this work: operations research and, more recently, field-based situation analysis.

Operations research studies apply formal analytic techniques, usually in small-scale settings, to examine the influence of particular elements of program activity (operations) on program outputs. Methods employed vary widely, from purely qualitative to randomized experiments. Over the years, operations research has contributed to the evolution of a number of differentiated program strategies (Ross and Frankenberg 1993), including:

- *Clinic-based services.* Services are offered at a fixed service delivery point, such as a maternity or health center.
- *Outreach and community-based distribution programs.* These programs are intended to contact populations beyond the reach of fixed clinics and health centers.
- *Social marketing.* This program distributes contraceptives (and in recent years other basic health inputs, such as iodized salts, vitamin A supplements, condoms for AIDS prevention, and the like) at subsidized prices through existing retail markets.
- *Postpartum programs.* These activities focus on the provision of family planning information and services to women during their prenatal visits and within one month to six weeks following delivery.

The mix, scale, and objectives of these basic strategies take different forms across various settings. Operations research has been useful in assessing relative effectiveness, although the limitations of method and scale (few large-scale programs are subject to systematic process observation) limit the generalizability of results and findings. At the same time, however, the wide dissemination of operations research efforts (primarily through externally financed grants and technical assistance) has been a major vehicle for building skills in program analysis in a number of settings (see Wawer and others 1991 for a review of experience in Sub-Saharan Africa).

In recent years, *situation analysis* methods have been developed to provide direct, comprehensive, and objective measures of program input and output at the level of individual service delivery points (such as the health center or family planning clinic). Situation analysis studies combine quantitative and qualitative methods, including direct observation, focus groups, interviews, sampling techniques, and small surveys to collect and analyze data on indicators measuring the availability and use of training and information, education, and communication programs; the level and functional quality of each of these systems; and the quality of services delivered by providers and clients' perceptions of this quality. Reflecting the growing interest in the application of managerial innovations such as "total quality management" to the health and family planning fields, considerable effort has been given to the development and dissemination of guidelines for "situation analysis" (see Fisher and others 1992) and their use to enhance client orientation and involvement in the quality of service at the country level. Recent applications have been useful in revealing how gaps in basic elements of service quality (unsympathetic provider attitude, absence of aseptic technique in clinical settings, missing commodities and equipment, and so forth) contribute to low service utilization and the failure to accept family planning services (see Mensch and others 1994).[3]

There are advantages and disadvantages to the use of these methods to study program process. Neither operations research nor situation analyses can be used to assess the effectiveness of a family planning program, and they often fail to identify or address the institutional or political variables that influence the quality of program implementation. At the same time, both methods are useful devices for engendering a "learning culture" within family planning implementation agencies, and the results of situation analyses have been important to an understanding of the significant role that service quality plays in influencing service utilization. Moreover, the collaborative style used in implementing such studies has enhanced the utilization of field observations in the formulation of program plans and policies. In Zimbabwe, for example, a situation analysis of rural health posts and their staff members revealed that most family planning service providers lacked sufficient counseling skills and demonstrated inadequate knowledge of several major forms of contraceptives. Study findings, prepared by a team including staff members from the family planning agency, were directly incorporated into a revision of the national family planning strategy upon study completion (World Bank, forthcoming).

Family Planning Performance Index

Interest in cross-national comparisons of population policy and programs developed early in the history of family planning research. In 1972, Lapham and Mauldin suggested that fifteen key items could be used to compare country experiences. and they presented data on these indicators for twenty countries. In 1976 these items were used by Berelson and Freedman in a study that included an additional twenty-three countries,[4] and in 1978 they were used by Mauldin and Berelson to analyze the fertility decline in ninety-four countries in 1965–75. Partially in response to the research needs of the 1984 *World Development Report*, the list of items was revised and the data updated to 1982 (Mauldin and Lapham 1983). The index that emerged from these efforts is known as the *family planning program performance index* (FPPI). It has since been updated twice, in 1989 and 1994 (Mauldin and Ross 1991; Mauldin 1995). The index characterizes program effort according to *policy and stage-setting activities,* or the activities that government and private agencies might undertake to affect the organization and implementation of a program; *service and service-related activities*, including the steps taken to make it easy for households to obtain and use a variety of family planning methods; *record-keeping and evaluation*; and the *availability and accessibility* of fertility control supplies and services, made possible by the first three components.

---

3. A recent methodological response to increasing demands for more timely feedback on program implementation is the development of methods for "Rapid Epidemiological Assessment" and "Rapid Anthropological Assessment" (see Smith 1989 and Scrimshaw and Hurtado 1987 for an overview of proposed methods). No reports on the application of these methods in field settings have yet been formally published.

4. This round of scoring was used to analyze the performance of the Bank in the population field by an External Advisory Panel in the mid-1970s.

Outcome Evaluation

Outcome evaluations of family planning programs examine the programs' influence on contraceptive prevalence (percentage of married women of reproductive age using contraception) and on their long-term impact on fertility.[5] Such an evaluation requires that researchers establish how fertility would have changed in the absence of programs, or to differentiate the effects of socioeconomic changes on fertility from those attributable to programs.

Cross-national data for such evaluations have been available only since the late 1970s and early 1980s. Nevertheless, small-scale outcome evaluation efforts using experimental models were conducted and contributed to the development of programs as early as the mid-1970s. For example, the Narangwal Project, a large field experiment conducted in India between 1969 and 1974, showed the effectiveness of family planning services that are integrated with basic health care (Kielman and others 1983; Taylor and others 1983). The Narangwal Project also produced several important methodological innovations, including methods that allow researchers to account for the amount of time field workers spend on particular forms of service delivery and to estimate service contact coverage rates by category of service. In Bangladesh, the Matlab Demonstration Project was designed as a field experiment to evaluate the effects of improved availability, quality, and access in family planning services in a "low demand" social setting (Bhatia and others 1980). This project demonstrated that intensive family planning programs can effectively increase contraceptive prevalence in settings of low socioeconomic status where large families are desired. Just as significantly, the Matlab Project established one of the few experimental settings and sites in the world for prospective, longitudinal measurement of household status, program characteristics, and demographic responses.

Field experiments in several other settings, including the Danfa Project in rural Ghana and the Jamkhed Project in Maharashtra State in India, added to the growing body of evidence that family planning programs contributed to fertility decline. Reviews of the results of these projects served to strengthen arguments for increasing governmental and donor support for family planning and primary health care programs (see Cuca and Pierce 1977; Gwatkin and others 1980; Faruqee 1982; and Boulier 1985). But differences in methodology and the design of "treatment" interventions, combined with the concern that the process of developing and supervising an intensive demonstration project might create upward bias in results through a "halo" effect, made it difficult to generalize from the results.

A large body of cross-national studies that examine the effectiveness of family planning programs complement the experimental literature. Studies of this kind became feasible following the development and implementation of a major comparative study of world fertility and with the later development of the demographic and health status surveys.[6] These data, combined with the

---

5. Formally, contraceptive prevalence is an output, and fertility the outcome, of interest. Fertility data, however, are rarely collected on a routine basis at local levels through vital registration. As a consequence, many monitoring and evaluation systems, and much research, tend to treat contraceptive prevalence as an outcome variable. Srinivasan (1993) forcefully argues that this tendency undermines the validity of family planning measurements. A recent demonstration project in Indonesia shows that using actual birth data to target programs and focus community participation can increase the visibility, acceptance, and effectiveness of child health as well as family planning interventions.

6. These large-scale surveys produced comparable data sets on family planning, immunization, and maternal and child health care beginning in the early 1980s. Data are now available for fifty-one countries. Repeat surveys have been conducted at three- and five-year intervals in nineteen countries.

FPPI, enabled the development of a series of cross-national regression analyses of the relationships among socioeconomic changes, family planning programs, and fertility effects. A review of these studies conducted as background to the 1984 *World Development Report* on Population and Development (World Bank 1984a) concluded that improvements in the performance of family planning programs are associated with greater declines in fertility. The review also estimated the effect of family planning programs net of fertility reductions attributable to earlier trends in fertility and socioeconomic changes. The report concluded that between 1965 and 1975, "for a hypothetical country experiencing the average increases in literacy, urbanization, life expectancy and income per capita over the decade" and attaining an average score on family planning level of effort in the early 1970s, "33 percent of the fertility decline is attributable to fertility reduction prior to 1965, only 27 percent to the direct effects of socioeconomic change, and fully 40 percent to family planning effort" (Boulier 1983).

The conclusion that family planning contributes to fertility decline has not gone undisputed. In a particularly influential reexamination of much of the same data that led others to this positive conclusion, Pritchett (1994) concluded that "the level of 'unmet need' and other measures of contraceptive access are not empirically important determinants of fertility." He argued that *unmet need* does not reflect only women who want contraceptives, but also those who require motivation to want what they need. A large portion of measured unmet need also represents women who are currently pregnant or otherwise infecund, and a substantial number of women who wish to alter the spacing of their births rather than to limit overall family size. Pritchett's critique has encouraged a reexamination of the concept of unmet need and has created renewed interest in the determinants of demand side variables, including desired family size and marriage age (influenced by socioeconomic elements such as the level of women's education).

Studies of Efficiency and Cost-Effectiveness

Although family planning programs have been subjected to voluminous evaluation, few evaluations include the data on program costs required for an analysis of the cost-effectiveness of particular program elements. There is considerable agreement on the validity of the FPPI, but very little work has been done to disaggregate the relative effectiveness of each of the indicators of program strength in the index or to estimate the costs of strengthening individual elements of program performance in selected settings. In part, these difficulties stem from the problems of assembling standardized cost data for family planning programs across sites and studies (Buckner and others 1995). Some studies have been done, however, including an examination of the impact and cost-effectiveness of contraceptive methods in Colombia (Janowitz and Bratt 1994); an assessment of the effectiveness and cost-effectiveness of postpartum family planning service provision (the IUD) in Peru (Foreit and others 1993); a study of the cost-effectiveness of five alternative service delivery methods for providing voluntary surgical contraception in Guatemala (McBride and others 1987); a cost-benefit analysis of the family planning program in Mexico (Nortman and others 1986); a study of the cost-effectiveness of the Family Planning Health Services Project in Matlab, Bangladesh (Simmons and others 1991); and an examination of the cost-effectiveness and financial efficiency of the PROFAMILIA Female Sterilization Program in Colombia (Williams and others 1990). All of the studies highlight the importance of the frequency and quality of client-provider relations in the success of a program (see box 3.1), but none enables a more generalized estimate of the marginal costs of introducing particular program elements in a given setting.

Box 3.1: Elements of Effective Family Planning Programs

A recent World Bank paper on family planning programs reviewed the large and growing body of results to identify what makes programs effective (Bulatao 1993). Several central elements of effectiveness were identified:

Accessibility
Successful programs provide access to a wide range of contraceptive methods and facilitate their continued use. An important associated element that affects program success is the availability of a variety of methods to meet the needs of women and families at different stages of their reproductive lives.

Assuring quality
Successful programs provide counseling and information on the potential side effects of the contraceptives considered and demonstrate respect for client social and religious sensibilities. Sharp social, religious, or class differences between provider and consumer reduce consumer satisfaction and can lead to high dropout rates and less effective programs.

Promotional activities
(Also referred to as information, education, and communication, or IEC)
Promotional activities play a major role in the delivery of family planning services, although it has been difficult to develop empirical evidence of the effectiveness of particular approaches and campaigns. Both mass media and face-to-face methods have been successfully employed, but face-to-face methods appear to be the most potent.

Effective program management
This element focuses on ensuring that contraceptive distribution and logistics systems are functional, that staff are well trained in the clinical aspects of service delivery and client relations, and that resources are available and managed at the appropriate levels of the delivery system. Decentralized managerial structures enhance accountability and responsiveness to consumer demand at the local level.

Assessing Family Planning Evaluation Literature

The evaluative literature on the effectiveness of family planning programs is relatively dense. In-depth analyses based on experimental, national, and cross-national surveys provide substantial evidence that deliberate family planning programs contribute to reduced fertility, although the pace and degree of progress is influenced by a variety of socioeconomic factors. The methods employed to develop this evidence appear to be broadly appropriate, although the FPPI is based on subjective judgments developed by a small number of expert observers. Estimation of the levels and trends in contraceptive prevalence and total fertility rates is based on data collected through well-designed and carefully implemented national surveys that have been subjected to rigorous methodological review before implementation. Although uncertainties remain about the magnitude of their contribution, there is strong evidence that family planning programs do contribute to reduced fertility. Considerable consensus on the elements of successful family planning programs has emerged from a growing body of process studies of program implementation. This literature has been particularly useful in highlighting the importance of service quality in determining participation levels and continued use of contraceptive methods. Evaluations of the relative strengths and weaknesses of alternative organizational and managerial structures for service delivery are less frequent, and their findings less convincing. The suggestion that organizational structures match the local institutional and managerial environments is a useful generalization that can be gleaned from this literature.

Evaluating Health Policies and Programs

A large body of theoretical and empirical work addresses the evaluation of health policies and programs. Relevant studies cover a wide array of issues, ranging from evaluations of the clinical efficacy of drugs and medical procedures to analyses of the impact of macroeconomic adjustment on public health services. The literature evaluating programs and policies in developing countries, while extensive, is seriously constrained by the limited availability of timely and reliable measures of mortality and morbidity in the majority of developing countries.[7] Not surprisingly, given these conditions, the materials reviewed for this study were found to be long on theoretical and methodological prescription and short on field-level implementation and empirical results.

This section concentrates on studies that have actually been undertaken and only indirectly refers to theoretical discussions of potentially useful methods for program evaluation. The review covers four major groups of studies: evaluations of the effectiveness of specific interventions; evaluations of the effectiveness of large-scale programs or delivery systems as a whole; studies of the mortality impact of health interventions; and studies on the relative cost-effectiveness of health interventions. Studies conducted to establish the biological or clinical efficacy of particular procedures (such as vaccines and specific contraceptive methods) are not covered. These would be more appropriately considered in the context of an evaluation of health research.[8]

Disease-Specific Interventions

The first major class of evaluation studies assess the impact of specific interventions on a given disease or condition. Most of the studies employ a combination of methods but ideally are randomized, controlled field trials examining the incidence of an intervention on mortality, case-fatality rates, and the incidence and prevalence of the disease in a selected population. Where clinical trials assess biological efficacy at the individual level, these studies try to assess *epidemiological efficacy* for a population. The effectiveness of particular interventions is not always easy to establish because other influences, such as method of delivery, can intrude. Oral rehydration therapy administered by trained staff in carefully controlled field trials, for example, may prove more effective than the same therapy administered by mothers. Moreover, cost and ethical considerations often result in the introduction of multiple interventions in a single setting, further complicating efforts to interpret the findings. These considerations render the literature

---

7. Coverage for vital statistics (based on civil registration of births, deaths, and marriages) on crude birth is about 99 percent in developed countries and Eastern Europe, but less than 1 percent in Sub-Saharan Africa, 22 percent in the Middle East and North Africa, 43 percent in Latin America, and 10 percent in Asia. India and China both have limited systems for sample registration (covering about 10 million households in China and only representative at the district level and above in India). The absence of adequate vital data is the most fundamental constraint on the development of systems to monitor and evaluate health outcomes, but this problem has never been addressed in Bank lending in the sector.

8. Nevertheless, as articulated in a recent report (Commission on Health Research for Development 1990), expenditures on such studies can be considered a public good, and gaps in capacity to conduct such research in developing countries need to be addressed.

on the major interventions generally included in the concept of "primary health care" large and complex.

The World Bank's preparations for *Investing in Health*, the 1993 *World Development Report*, included a compilation of data from the epidemiological literature on the effectiveness of fifty of the most important public health and clinical health interventions (see Jamison and others 1993). The work was completed as a necessary first step in the completion of the Bank's analysis of disease control priorities and includes comprehensive reviews of the effectiveness literature for a wide range of disease-specific interventions.[9] Table 3.1 summarizes the results of a cost-effectiveness analysis for two groups of interventions.[10] *Public health* interventions are directed to or sought by entire populations or population subgroups, whereas *clinical* interventions are usually directed to individuals in health centers and large hospitals.

The studies have produced two noteworthy findings that have affected thinking on the design and delivery of health care systems. First, clinical and public health interventions are often relatively inexpensive, which suggests that both should be made available in local settings to get the greatest return for the money spent—a dramatic shift from the long-held assumption that community-based primary care services could be effective, even in the absence of clinical services. Second, many of the most cost-effective interventions require significant *behavioral changes* at the household level (such as breastfeeding, condom use, smoking cessation, and use of iodized salt). This suggests that many of the most cost-effective health interventions are more a matter of promotion and communication than medical care, which has clear implications for the design of delivery systems. Traditional medical models of health status change may not always be adequate and must be revamped to incorporate efforts to change the way consumers (and providers) think and behave. Included in the paradigm will be information about the determinants of disease and health-seeking behaviors.

Evaluation of Impact of Health Programs

Assessing the effectiveness of a single, disease-specific intervention is relatively straightforward because the data—for example, on the incidence of the disease and its mortality rate—are not difficult to distinguish. Few programs can afford to address a single specific condition to the exclusion of other health problems, however, and many health problems are likely to benefit from multiple interventions. Assessing the effectiveness of such a program is difficult. For instance, an initiative to prevent diarrheal disease is likely to employ a combination

---

9. Rashad, Gray, and Boerma (1995) also provide a compendium of analyses of the impact of particular disease interventions. Since most of the findings are more detailed expositions of those presented in Jamison and others (1993), these materials are not reviewed here.

10. Readers are referred to the disease-specific chapters in Jamison and others (1993) for a more in-depth discussion of the evidence on costs and effectiveness for each intervention.

Table 3.1: Intervention Characteristics and Cost-Effectiveness

Potential intervention	Strategy	Objective application	Potential	Age group[a]
$25 per DALY[b]				
Breastfeeding promotion	Public health: Behavior change	Secondary prevention	Moderate	Childhood
Diphtheria-pertussis-tetanus plus polio immunization	Public health: Immunization	Primary prevention	Substantial	Childhood
Measles immunization	Public health: Immunization	Primary prevention	Substantial	Childhood
Tuberculosis immunization	Public health: Immunization	Primary prevention	Moderate	Childhood
Iodization of salt	Public health: Mass chemoprophylaxis	Secondary prevention	Substantial	All ages
Fortification of sugar with vitamin A	Public health: Mass chemoprophylaxis	Secondary prevention	Substantial	Childhood
Semiannual mass dose of vitamin A	Public health: Mass chemoprophylaxis	Secondary prevention	Substantial	Childhood
Rotavirus immunization	Public health: Immunization	Primary prevention	Limited	Childhood
Hepatitis B immunization	Public health: Immunization	Primary prevention	Substantial	Childhood
Medical treatment of measles with vitamin A	Clinical: Primary care	Cure	Limited	Childhood
Medical treatment of acute respiratory infections with antibiotics	Clinical: Primary care	Cure	Moderate	Childhood
Use of ophthalmic ointment at birth to prevent gonococcal infection	Clinical: Primary care	Primary prevention	Substantial	Childhood
Targeted mass anthelmintics	Public health: Mass chemoprophylaxis	Secondary prevention	Substantial	School age
Antituberculosis chemotherapy with short-course hospitalization	Clinical: District hospital	Cure	Substantial	All ages
Smoking prevention or cessation programs	Public health: Behavior change	Primary prevention plus secondary prevention	Substantial	Adults
Use of condoms to prevent excess births and sexually transmitted diseases	Public health: Behavior change	Primary prevention	Moderate	Adults
Blood screening for HIV	Clinical: District hospital, referral hospital	Primary prevention	Limited	Adults
Iodine injections for pregnant women	Public health: Mass chemoprophylaxis	Secondary prevention	Substantial	Adults
Daily oral iron for pregnant women	Public health: Mass chemoprophylaxis	Secondary prevention	Limited	Adults
Cataract removal	Clinical: District hospital	Cure	Substantial	Elderly
Medical treatment of leprosy	Clinical: Primary care	Cure	Moderate	Adults
Malaria control with chemical pesticides	Public health: Environmental	Primary prevention	Moderate	All ages
$25–$75 per DALY				
Pneumococcal immunization	Public health: Immunization	Primary prevention	Moderate	All ages
Use of oral rehydration solutions	Public health: Behavior change	Secondary prevention	Substantial	School age
Improved weaning practices	Public health: Behavior change	Secondary prevention	Moderate	Childhood
Food supplements for children	Public health: Mass chemoprophylaxis	Secondary prevention	Limited	School age
Food supplements for pregnant women	Public health: Mass chemoprophylaxis	Secondary prevention	Limited	Adults
Improved antenatal care by upgrading facilities and providing family planning	Clinical: Primary care, district hospital, referral hospital	Primary prevention	Limited	Adults
$75–$250 per DALY				
Medical treatment of tetanus	Clinical: District hospital	Cure	Limited	Childhood
Cholera immunization	Public health: Immunization	Primary prevention	Limited	Childhood

Table 3.1 (Continued)

Potential intervention	Strategy	Objective application	Potential	Age group[a]
Malaria control with passive case finding and chemical pesticides with treatment	Clinical: Primary care, public health, environmental	Primary prevention plus cure	Moderate	All ages
Medical and surgical treatment of leprosy complications	Clinical: Primary care, district hospital	Rehabilitation plus palliation	Limited	All ages
Antibiotic prophylaxis for children with history of rheumatic fever	Clinical: Primary care	Secondary prevention	Limited	Childhood
Public preventive package for most cardiovascular risk factors	Public health: Behavior change	Primary prevention plus secondary prevention	Moderate	Adults
Insulin therapy for non–insulin-dependent diabetic individuals	Clinical: Primary care	Secondary prevention	Limited	Adults, elderly
Management of stable angina with medication	Clinical: Primary care	Rehabilitation plus secondary prevention	Limited	Adults, elderly
Management of post-myocardial infarction or post-stroke patients	Clinical: Primary care, public health, behavior change	Secondary prevention	Moderate	Adults, elderly
Low-cost medical management of unstable or myocardial infarction	Clinical: District hospital	Rehabilitation plus secondary prevention	Limited	Adults, elderly
Cancer pain management	Clinical: Primary care	Palliation	Substantial	All ages
Onchocerciasis control with chemical pesticides	Public health: Environmental	Primary prevention	Moderate	All ages
Schizophrenia or manic-depressive illness treatment with medication	Clinical: Primary care	Rehabilitation	Moderate	Adults
$250–$1,000 per DALY				
Referral of pharyngitis cases for antibiotic prophylaxis to prevent rheumatic fever and rheumatic heart disease	Public health: Screening and referral	Primary prevention	Limited	Childhood
Improved dengue case management through education of health care providers	Clinical: Behavior change	Primary prevention	Limited	All ages
>$1,000 per DALY				
Medical and surgical management of chronic obstructive pulmonary disease	Clinical: Referral hospital	Rehabilitation plus palliation	Limited	Adults, elderly
Surgery for rheumatic heart disease	Clinical: Referral hospital	Rehabilitation plus secondary prevention	Limited	Adults
Management of moderate hypertension with medication	Clinical: Primary care	Secondary prevention	Moderate	Adults, elderly
Management of hypercholesterolemia with medication	Clinical: Primary care	Secondary prevention	Limited	Adults, elderly
High-cost management of myocardial infarction or unstable angina	Clinical: District hospital	Secondary prevention	Limited	Adults, elderly
Management of coronary artery disease with surgery	Clinical: Referral hospital	Rehabilitation plus secondary prevention	Limited	Adults, elderly
Medical and surgical management of cancers	Clinical: Referral hospital	Cure plus palliation	Limited	All ages
Dengue control with chemical pesticides, with or without improved case management	Public health: Environmental	Primary prevention	Moderate	All ages
Dengue control by drainage and land management, with or without improved case management	Public health: Environmental	Primary prevention	Limited	All ages

a. Age groups are defined as follows: childhood = age 0 to 4; school age = age 5 to 14; adults = age 15 to 59; elderly = age 60 plus. Most interventions will be useful for a range of age groups; the principal age group served by an intervention is indicated.
b. DALY = disability-adjusted life-year.
Source: Jamison and others (1993).

of interventions, including the promotion of sanitation, clean water supplies, and oral rehydration therapy. These evaluations must then determine the contribution of each intervention to the program's overall success.

The process is further complicated by the lack of agreement on a single best measure or index of health status. While mortality may immediately seem the most obvious indicator, mortality at different ages and among varied social groups has differing social and individual welfare weights. Mortality data, which do not indicate changes in morbidity or disability, are not a feasible measure for many programs, for several reasons. First, assembling reliable baseline information on mortality status requires special surveys because few countries have reliable or generalizable vital registration systems. Experience with such survey methods has not been encouraging. Among the tools needed, retrospective autopsies are expensive, and retrospective reports of mortality at the household level are subject to measurement error. In addition, controlling for secular trends in mortality can be problematic, and sample size requirements for estimating change in mortality (a rare event) can be prohibitively expensive, even when they are accurately estimated.[11] Experimental approaches require costly administrative controls and supervision. In the Narangwal Project (Taylor and others 1983), one of the few large-scale multi-intervention field experiments, the costs to establish and maintain the data for the experiment amounted to about 40 percent of the costs of service delivery (Faruqee 1985).

Measuring the Burden of Disease

Investing in Health (World Bank 1993) responded to this challenge with the concept of a disability-adjusted life-year (DALY). The DALY is an indicator of the time lived with a disability and the time lost to premature mortality. The duration of time lost is calculated using estimates of life expectancy, and streams of time are discounted at 3 percent (Murray and others 1994). Unhealthy life-years are given lower weights than healthy years, depending on degree of disability. The effectiveness of interventions to address morbidity or disability can then be compared with interventions to avert mortality (Jamison and others 1993). Use of the DALY has clear advantages over using mortality alone. It explicitly accounts for age differences in mortality, and it includes disability, and thus morbidity or illness, in its definition. It also adds a time dimension to the measurement of death. Analysis of the distribution of DALYs in a population, which can be done by estimating causes of death, morbidity, and age and sex characteristics, enable estimation of the burden of disease which can therefore be treated as the outcome of interest. The major advantage of using DALYs to estimate the burden of disease is that they provide an integrated, comprehensive method of capturing the average amount of ill health (morbidity and mortality) that will be experienced over a lifetime and serve as a common measure for evaluating priorities among a large number of causes of death and disability (Murray and others 1994). Despite this step forward, estimating the burden of disease at the country level is an onerous, data-intensive task, and such estimates are only now being prepared. These estimates are not yet sufficiently robust to enable impact evaluation of health programs. As national capacity to estimate the burden of disease is developed, it may become feasible to use burden-of-disease data as a basis for assessing program impact, but this will not be possible within the next five to ten years.

---

11. If the baseline infant mortality rate is, for example, 140 per 1,000 live births, and the intervention is expected to reduce mortality by 10 percent, baseline and follow-up surveys would need to cover 14,450 live births to provide an 80 percent chance of finding a significant difference at the 95 percent level (Rashad and others 1995). The situation for assessing changes in the maternal mortality ratio, typically estimated in developing countries at 4.5 per 1,000 live births, is, of course, even more demanding.

Not surprisingly, satisfactory evaluation designs for the measurement of the effectiveness of large-scale programs are rare. While it is possible to establish the efficacy of a single intervention in small-scale, tightly controlled settings, it is methodologically difficult to evaluate the effectiveness of large-scale, multi-intervention programs. Establishing longitudinal surveillance systems and experimental sites analogous to the Matlab Project in Bangladesh may be one solution (the World Bank is currently funding such a project in Indonesia). It may also be worth considering whether large, multi-intervention programs should be replaced with a series of more manageable and deliberately designed learning efforts.

Delivery Systems

In response to the difficulties inherent in evaluating health services by measuring outcomes, much of the literature focuses on measuring particular health outputs. Many output measures are used in evaluation, depending on the intervention or range of interventions to be assessed (for instance, the number of immunizations in a program to expand immunizations, or the number of case-years of protection for a parasitic disease control program). But output measures specific to each intervention cannot be used to compare different interventions or to estimate the overall effectiveness of a program of interventions.

Service Utilization. One alternative that has attracted considerable attention is a more general measure of output, such as the utilization rate of a given service. Utilization reviews are not equivalent to a study of an intervention's impact—a service can be heavily used with little or no measurable effect on mortality or morbidity. While utilization studies can disguise important dimensions of effectiveness, such as service quality, they can also reveal whether the necessary inputs are reaching the intended target group and offer useful insights into the demand for services.

A recent exercise to determine health policy research priorities emphasized the importance of further examinations of service utilization as a measure of need, equity, and resource allocation issues in developing countries (Gish 1995). Reviews of the effects of quality and demand in health programs further reinforces the potential usefulness of utilization as an indicator of program effectiveness.

The Role of Quality. Another approach to evaluating the delivery of health services probes the elements that lead to consumer satisfaction with service provision and quality. For instance, interviews with heads of household in two rural villages in Sri Lanka examined the use and evaluation (satisfaction) of health care services. The study found that in one village members of female-headed households used services more frequently than members of families headed by males. The study found that characteristics such as age, marital status, and education affected women's use and evaluation of health services. Education was not associated with securing immunizations by the majority of families (Wickrama and Keith 1990).

Process studies have also been used to identify ways to improve the utilization of services. For example, in the Idjwi district of Zaire, where health centers are supported by the sale of drugs but have had low utilization rates and high costs, the cost of visits was reduced by stabilizing the price of drugs and prescriptions. The study showed that despite a real price decrease of 20 percent, utilization of medical care did not improve, and the reduction in revenues led to deficits in most centers. The study hypothesized that the price decrease may not have been sufficient to produce changes in utilization, and that not enough time had elapsed (eight months) for any changes to become noticeable. In a neighboring area where the drugs are subsidized through donor assistance, utilization rates for curative care were twice as high as in Idjwi. "Therefore, if drugs are less expensive, the use of health services does improve" (Courtois and Dumoulin 1995, p. 185).

In Sri Lanka, an analysis of data for health facilities in four districts focused on costs in the public and private sectors. The study found, not surprisingly, that unit costs are extremely sensitive to utilization, and that unit costs for inpatient services in basic facilities are considerably higher than in complex facilities. The private sector provides a substantially different product than the public sector in both physical amenities (more floor space) and level of inputs (more personnel for each patient, with a different mix of providers). At the level of the basic hospital, the private sector delivers these amenities at a lower cost than the public sector. The payoff for introducing innovations in the public sector to reduce costs, increase the quality of inpatient services, and manage overcrowding in some heavily used facilities is potentially high. As the study concludes, "there are clear opportunities for more effective use of resources, especially through consolidating and rethinking the delivery of basic hospital and outpatient services in this country" (Griffin and others 1994, p. 5).

User Charges and Demand for Services. Other tools have been developed to study service delivery. Studies of the demand for services analyze the potential for introducing user charges to recover the costs of services. A recent review of these studies identified the following consistencies across a number of studies (Makinen and Raney 1994):

- Price influences the sick person's decision to use a health service, but not a great deal.
- Price influences the choice of provider more than the decision of whether to use services at all.
- Nonprice costs of using services (such as time and transportation) borne by consumers influence both the decision to use services and the choice of provider.
- People's perceptions of the quality of services (especially the availability of drugs) influence both the decision to use services and the choice of provider.
- Poor people often spend 5 percent or more of their incomes on health services.

The review also identified some inconsistent findings:

- Poor people are more sensitive to prices than their wealthier neighbors when choosing whether to use health services.
- Nonprice costs borne by consumers are more important than prices in choosing whether and what provider to use.

Whether households benefit from government expenditures on health care depends on the quality of the services delivered and how households respond to that quality. Recent research by Alderman and Lavy (1996), based on household surveys, show that consumers, even those in low-income households, are willing to pay fees for better health care if the fees translate into improved access and reliability. The paper confirms that quality factors (such as availability of drugs, number of nurses and doctors, existence of electricity, and water) have large and significant effects on demand; part of the change reflects shifts from the private sector to the public sector, and part represents a shift from self-care to the modern health sector. The results strongly suggest that if prices for public health services were raised and the revenues used to increase the quality of care, the use of both public and modern health care in general might in fact increase.

In addition to these studies, there are numerous country-level reports measuring the outputs of particular interventions. Advice and comparative discussions concerning particular programs—for instance, immunization programs or alternative approaches to the treatment of tuberculosis—are available but are of limited use in examining the performance of a health system as a whole. (The FPPI, discussed earlier, is the most highly developed of these schemes.) Suggestions and proposed methods for measuring outputs vary with the intervention and are most highly developed in the field of immunization, where there is considerable agreement on ideal immunization schedules, well-defined target age groups, and an increasingly adaptable technology (the thirty-household cluster survey) for estimating coverage rates in small populations. Unfortunately, at both international and national levels, advocates of individual interventions tend to reject output measurement systems that are useful for tracking a group of interventions, undermining efforts to target and track coverage of a broader package of health care interventions.

Value for Money in Health

Measures of cost-effectiveness, such as the DALY and accurate estimates of the total burden of disease at regional and national levels, provide a framework for more rational health planning. Various operational units of the Bank are currently working to incorporate these tools into the economic analysis of proposed projects. For example, Ravicz and others (1996) recently employed a participatory approach to estimating the burden of disease in Tanzania, Uganda, Kenya, Eritrea, and Uganda and to engage local policymakers in a review of the cost-effectiveness of their health expenditures. But such a method, while useful in stimulating dialogue about the relative effectiveness of health measures, is less useful in the consideration of larger questions of sectoral policy, such as the relative roles of government and the private sector in financing and providing even the most cost-effective package of interventions. These questions require a mix of institutional analysis and understanding of public choice issues which are beyond the scope of epidemiological and demographic methods.

There are additional limits to the use of cost-effectiveness to evaluate health policy choices. Interventions vary in their *specificity* (the proportion of recipients who will benefit, assuming that the intervention is applied exactly as it should be to all who should receive it), the degree to which they can be targeted to populations at risk, the variance in risk patterns across populations, and the level of compliance that can be expected with the "regimen" of the treatment (alternatively, in demand when a service is not epidemiologically or medically necessary). Because each of these variables is subject to economic, cultural, and managerial factors unrelated to the intervention itself, the cost effectiveness of the same intervention can vary (sometimes quite widely) within and between settings and population groups. Cost-effectiveness recommendations need to be filtered through analyses of the context and performance of specific delivery systems.

Unfortunately, one finds little in the literature that enables a broad characterization of the performance of the health care delivery system that is roughly analogous to the FPPI. Comparative studies of health systems are few and largely indeterminate, as described by Schieber (1995) for Organization for Economic Cooperation and Development (OECD) countries. The data requirements for making comparative judgments are enormous. Even policymakers who are able to agree on the most cost-effective package of services at the national level face the complex question of determining how best to ensure that the interventions are delivered.

Elements of Effective Health Service Delivery Programs

Given the complexities of measuring the effectiveness of health service delivery programs, it is perhaps not surprising that no body of literature or widely accepted measurement tool is available and that little empirical evidence on effective delivery systems can be found. Nevertheless, a considerable body of normative literature on the characteristics of effective delivery systems has recently become available. The World Bank's *Investing in Health* (1993) reviewed much of the prescriptive literature on how best to deliver both public health and clinical interventions. The report makes two broad suggestions for health policy that are of direct relevance to the design and potential effectiveness of alternative service delivery systems. First, it identifies the most cost-effective public health interventions:

- expanded immunization programs, defined to include micronutrient supplementation;
- school health programs to treat worm infections and micronutrient deficiencies and to provide health education;
- programs to increase public knowledge about family planning, nutrition, self-treatments. cues to seek care, and vector control and disease surveillance activities;
- programs to reduce consumption of tobacco, alcohol, and drugs;
- AIDS prevention programs with a strong component on sexually transmitted diseases (STDs).

Second, the report lists the most cost-effective clinical interventions, which it recommends as the "minimum package of essential clinical services" for which governments everywhere should ensure access and ensure efficient delivery. The list included the following:

- short-course chemotherapy for tuberculosis;
- management of the sick child;
- prenatal and delivery care;
- family planning;
- treatment of STDs;
- limited curative care (assessment, advice, alleviation of pain, and treatment of infection and minor trauma) and treatment of more complicated conditions as resources permit.

The report notes that governments can select from a group of instruments to ensure access and improve the efficiency of the program. It also identifies government actions that can be taken with regard to clinical services outside the essential package. The "minimum basic package" is remarkably similar to the list of interventions that have traditionally been identified with primary health care strategy.

The report suggests three strategies to make delivery systems more effective. First, it recommends a *structure* for service delivery: " a well-functioning district health system consisting of health posts and health centers as the first point of contact and district hospitals as referral facilities, with the two levels linked by emergency transport." Second, the report comments on the advantages and disadvantages of four alternative *sources of finance* for services—two private sources (out-of-pocket expenditures and voluntary insurance) and two public sources (compulsory insurance and government revenue). Third, the report discusses the advantages and disadvantages of three different forms of ownership—public, private, and nonprofit (the last two represent nongovernmental organizations, NGOs). Finally, the report builds on these elements to produce a set of suggested policies that governments could employ to improve the delivery of services (see table 3.2).

Table 3.2: Rationales and Directions for Government Action in the Finance and Delivery of Clinical Services

Area	Conditions that may call for government action: market failure and poverty	Directions for government action
Essential clinical services	Failure to treat, for example, tuberculosis and STDs creates risks for the general population. Public financing can help offset the additional external costs to society. Poor people have limited ability to save or borrow to meet unexpected and uninsured health expenses. Families, including children, can fall into poverty because of ill health.	*Finance* essential clinical services by reallocating current government spending. In low-income countries this may mean increasing public expenditures for health. *Require* through legislation that social insurance or mandated private insurance cover an essential package. *Encourage* more private and NGO provision of essential services, through appropriate legislation and targeted public subsidies.
Clinical services outside the essential package	In insurance markets, selection bias leads to lack of coverage for high-risk groups. "Moral hazard," by insulating patient and provider from the cost implications of their decisions, results in overuse of services. The asymmetry of information between patient and provider can cause suppliers to induce excess demand.	*Reduce or eliminate* subsidization of clinical services outside the essential package. Subsidies for public provision of services at less than cost and tax relief for employer and employee health insurance payments often cover services with low cost-effectiveness and primarily benefit the wealthy. *Legislate* compulsory social insurance or mandated private insurance or define the national essential package comprehensively. *Limit* government involvement in delivery of nonessential services and encourage competition in service delivery among government, NGOs, and the private sector. *Regulate* private insurance by, for example, requiring community risk rating and forbidding the rejection of high-risk consumers. *Define* the exact content of prepaid packages of care to serve as the products bought and sold in the insurance market. *Encourage* the use of prepayment or salary-based approaches to provider compensation. *Foster* improvements in the quality of private provision by encouraging self-regulation of hospitals, medical schools, and physicians and by disseminating performance indicators.

Source: "Investing in Health," World Development Report, 1993.

These suggestions, however, are not based on empirical reviews of the combinations of structure, ownership, and financing that are the most efficient or effective, nor do they provide guidance in managing transitions between one form of delivery and another. A more recent Bank policy study (Musgrove 1996) provides a more in-depth theoretical discussion of appropriate public and private roles in health and presents empirical information on how countries organize health financing and delivery and how these decision relate to a population's health status, the level of expenditure on health, and the consequences of these decisions for consumer satisfaction and medical and financial equity. The study concludes with a set of recommendations for what governments should and should not do to ensure equity and efficiency in the health market. A general observation that emerges is that governments have demonstrated a tendency to undervalue certain instruments (such as the capacity to mandate and regulate aspects of the market) and to rely excessively on the direct provision of services in response to health needs. The report provides an important normative basis for analyzing the likely effects of health sector reform initiatives. These policy suggestions have become central to the current discussions of health sector reform in the projected HNP portfolio.

Implications for Evaluation

What lessons can be gleaned from this diverse literature to add to our understanding of development effectiveness in the HNP sector and contribute to the design of HNP evaluations?

First, there is considerably greater clarity in the evaluation of family planning programs than there is in the evaluation of health policies and programs. One reason for this disparity is that family planning is a single "health intervention." There is much empirical work that can serve as the basis for more efficient and effective programs. Defining development effectiveness for a family planning program is relatively straightforward, although achieving it may not be.

The situation is much less clear in the case of health programs, largely because of the multidimensional nature of the outcome. Even if one overlooks the measurement difficulties, including secular trends in mortality and socioeconomic status, it is difficult to estimate the direct effects of health services on mortality because of the large number of programs that may be included within "health services." Recent efforts to refine definitions of outcome through the use of the DALY suffer from many of the same problems that damaged the "old" measurement of mortality. DALYs are equally difficult to measure and document, particularly with the lack of reliable systems for reporting birth and death that is typical of most developing countries. Improvements in *ex ante* decisionmaking on service priorities may indeed result from more widespread use of cost-effectiveness analysis in choosing the mix of interventions (health services), but they will be of limited utility in ex post evaluation for the same reasons that mortality is an inadequate tool.

Utilization and demand studies are useful in describing output patterns in the service delivery systems but do little to describe the systems themselves. They have not yet been employed in a comparative framework to test the empirical validity of recent assumptions on the most efficient and effective delivery systems (that is, combinations of source of finance, ownership, and structure) to reach selected subgroups, such as the rural and urban poor, in particular country settings.

Further work to define development effectiveness in the sector requires an effort to collect information on "who is using what provider for what service" to bear on the question of choices among alternative delivery systems. This would suggest that evaluation of HNP programs should start with an analysis of the relevance of delivery system design (covering structure and functional characteristics, financing, and forms of ownership) and comparisons of the utilization of services among delivery systems in order to assess relative efficiency and effectiveness.

4. Evaluations of HNP in the Bank

Twenty-five Years of Experience

The Bank's first initiatives in the HNP sector emerged in the late 1960s in response to the growing recognition of the challenge to economic development represented by rapid population growth. This concern, and international consensus that private and public sector family planning programs could influence fertility trends, led to the establishment of the Population Projects Department in 1969 and the development of World Bank research and analyses of population policy (King and others 1974 presents the Bank's first published population research and policy recommendations). The Population Projects Department led the preparation and appraisal of twenty-two loans to address the issue of population in South and East Asia and Latin America and four nutrition projects in Latin America. The population program was seen as an important element of the Bank's commitment to meeting basic human needs.

At the same time, the Bank was becoming increasingly concerned with mitigation of the negative health impact of investments in other sectors (for example, preventing the spread of schistosomiasis in areas altered by large-scale dam and irrigation projects). Work in this area was led and monitored by an Office of Environment and Health, which was also active in developing health components to complement rural development, agriculture, and infrastructure projects. Health policy had also begun to receive greater attention at the international level. In 1977, the World Health Organization (WHO) sponsored the Conference on Health for All by the Year 2000. This gathering served to formalize the consensus that health status in developing countries could and should be improved through the provision of low-cost primary health care services. The Bank was responsive to this interest. Following an initial statement of health sector policy in 1975 that included a determination not to lend directly for health, the Bank altered its policy in 1980 and initiated lending in the health sector. To accommodate this mandate, the Office of Environment and Health, with its health and nutrition specialists, and the Population Projects Department were merged to form the new Health, Nutrition, and Population Projects Department. Direct lending in the health sector was initiated.

Policy

In an initial attempt to set out a rationale for activity in the health sector, the Bank produced a *Health Sector Policy Paper* in 1975. The paper presented the justification for the decision not to lend directly for basic health services, but instead to concentrate on improving the health service components and limiting the potentially negative health consequences of projects in other sectors. Projects would continue to be justified by objectives other than health improvements alone. The rationale demonstrated the belief that health programs should not be isolated efforts, but part of a broad program of socioeconomic development designed to reduce mortality and fertility. It also reflected concerns about the feasibility of low-cost health care systems, the lack of *political will* to institute significant reforms, and uncertainties about the Bank's proper role in the health sector, especially in its relationship with the WHO.

Despite the decision to limit Bank operations in health to components of other projects, the 1975 report raised a number of concerns about the state of health service delivery in developing countries and the inefficiency and inequity of government spending for health. The paper argued that to increase the effectiveness of official health services and ensure more equitable access to care, governments must curtail their expenditures on hospitals and highly trained personnel. Greater gains in health would be realized by *improving health service delivery at the community level* by extending the coverage and responsiveness of the primary health care system and extending primary care into the community. Despite the importance of this agenda, the paper advised against direct lending for basic health services, largely because the Bank's role in health was uncertain, borrower governments appeared to lack the political commitment to reform, and such lending could imply a shift in emphasis away from family planning and population goals.

From 1975 through 1978, the Bank provided technical and financial assistance to forty-four countries for seventy health components of projects in other sectors. In addition, the Bank prepared seven health sector studies and several population sector studies and established working relationships with the WHO and other major agencies working in the health sector. This experience formed the basis for a significant change in the Bank's health policy stance in 1980.

Direct Lending for Basic Health Services

The *1980 Health Sector Policy Paper* committed the Bank to direct lending in the health sector. The paper identified activities for possible inclusion in health projects and outlined a policy that emphasized improvement in the context and circumstances of basic health care delivery. The major elements of the policy included the development of basic health infrastructure, the training of community health workers and paraprofessional staff, the strengthening of logistics and the supply of essential drugs, the provision of maternal and child health care, and improved family planning and disease control.

The change in policy was justified by four noteworthy points. First, the Bank possessed a capacity for programming and sectoral analysis that could be harnessed to support extension of national health care coverage, particularly primary health care, in developing countries. Second, a broader policy of lending for health was seen as an essential element of the Bank's commitment to alleviating poverty. Third, direct lending for health projects was viewed as necessary to complement and rationalize Bank activities in the health sector. And fourth, direct lending in health could serve as a vehicle for discussions of population issues and support of family planning services delivered through the health care system.

In 1975 the Bank had been very uncertain of its role in the health sector. By 1980 a new confidence had emerged with the commitment to improve and extend the coverage of basic health services in developing countries. The question of *political commitment* on the part of borrower countries remained, however, and the policy paper set out a number of criteria to inform Bank selection of countries and projects to be financed. These criteria included the willingness of a country to develop sectoral planning capacity and prepare long-term plans for more accessible basic services; the financial and institutional feasibility, cost-effectiveness, and replicability of the project; the social acceptance of the activities to be funded; the reliability and effectiveness of service delivery systems; and the capacity of government and the implementing institutions to absorb external assistance and finance recurrent costs following implementation of the project.

The Role of Government

In both the 1975 and 1980 documents, the rationale for government action in health, and for Bank support, was the prevalence of market failures in the provision and financing of health care and the need for more equitable distribution of services. The impetus for an expanded program in support of health within the Bank was the desire to create a basis of greater involvement to spur discussions of national health policies and programs and to permit the Bank to initiate considerations of the role of health in overall development. Initial operations were expected to stress the development of planning and management skills and the establishment of organizational structures and procedures for administration of health care systems.

Both the 1975 and 1980 policy papers critiqued public spending for health in developing countries; both documents also held that the most effective strategy to improve health was the revision of the administrative allocation of resources, with particular emphasis on the provision of services for the poorest groups in society. This generally meant direct delivery of services through facilities owned or operated by government and financed by general government revenues. While the role of private financing for health was duly acknowledged, the policy papers focused their attention on strategies for improving the effectiveness of government spending.

The central role of government action in reducing mortality and fertility was further reinforced in the 1984 *World Development Report, Population and Development*. The report presented a threefold policy message. First, rapid population growth is a development problem, inextricably bound up with questions of macroeconomic and sectoral stability. Second, public policy can play a role in reducing fertility. And third, experience shows that policy makes a difference.

A central theme presented in the report is the importance of public policy in encouraging people to have fewer children. The justification for government action is two fold. First, there is a gap between the private rewards and the social gains of having many children. It is considered appropriate for government to "narrow the gap between private and social perceptions . . .[and] act as custodians of society." Governments interested in social welfare "are meant to have longer time horizons than their individual constituents, and to weigh the interests of future generations against those of the present" (World Bank 1984a, p. 54). By developing a *social contract*, the government frees each individual couple from its "isolation paradox"; that is, from the need to decide on their own to have more children than they would want if there were a socially accepted policy in place limiting family size.

The second justification for government action to reduce fertility is the problem of "myopia" and lack of information. Without information, individuals and families make decisions about family size that fail to reflect changing societal conditions and preferences. By providing information on changing mortality and the health benefits of fertility control, government can encourage parents in their desire to have fewer children. "Government's role in developing and enhancing a *social contract* to lower fertility provides the basis for public subsidies to family planning" (World Bank 1984a, p. 56).

Reassessing the Role of Government

The 1987 policy study *Financing Health Services in Developing Countries: An Agenda for Reform* (World Bank 1987a) tackled one of the central policy themes identified in 1975 and 1980—inefficient and inequitable public spending in health and the ongoing problem of financing recurrent costs—but approached the issue from a very different starting point. The slow economic growth and record budget deficits in the 1980s dramatically affected public spending, prompting questions about the feasibility of increased public spending in health and possible alternative approaches to financing health care for future generations. The study argued that even in the absence of severe budget constraints, new approaches to the financing of health care are required in order to improve both the efficiency and the equity of health care. Four policies to reform government financing of health care were proposed: implementation of user charges at government health facilities, especially for drugs and curative care; introduction of insurance or other risk coverage to help mobilize resources for health while protecting households from large financial losses; more effective utilization of nongovernment resources, including nonprofit groups, private physicians, pharmacies, and other health practitioners; and introduction of decentralized planning, budgeting, and purchasing for government health services, particularly interventions that offer private benefits in exchange for a fee. While focusing on the prospects for improvements in the internal efficiency of health spending, these reforms also offered an opportunity for greater cooperation between the public and private sectors in providing and financing health care, particularly by making more effective use of the private sector to provide health services that extend essentially private benefits to the recipients.

The main implication of the 1987 study for the Bank's work in health lay in the nature and content of its policy dialogue with borrower governments. The report noted that "the Bank is now broadening that dialogue, both with borrowers and other lending agencies, to encourage consideration of new financing approaches to rethink prevailing strategies and the concepts on which they are based"(World Bank 1987a, p. 49). This broadening of the dialogue introduced questions not only about ways of improving the efficiency of financing arrangements in health but also about more fundamental considerations of the proper role for government in the health sector. Where the study stopped short was in providing the analytic tools needed to assess the appropriate role of government in the variety of fiscal and epidemiological contexts confronted in the developing world. In addition, little attention is given to the reasons for the current allocations of spending in the health sector and the institutional and incentive mechanisms that create a disparity between the actual distribution of resources and the expected configuration.

The Political Economy of Health

Two policy working papers, by Birdsall (1989) and Birdsall and James (1990), focused explicitly on the issue of public choice in health policy. They argued that the degree of efficiency and redistribution in public policymaking is endogenous and politically determined. Unlike the earlier "welfarist" models of government, these presentations argue that the political economy of public choice makes the inefficiencies and inequities of health services financed and provided by government inevitable. Drawing on the broader views of public choice theory, Birdsall argued that, in addition to the inadequacy of public resources in the majority of developing countries to address the growing complexity of biomedical realities, public officials inevitably serve their own interests more readily than the broader public interest. Political interest groups exert significant influence in the actual distribution of resources in the health sector. Power is ceded to such groups because of information asymmetries and uncertainty among policymakers, providers, and beneficiaries and the presence of bureaucratic management and financing systems with low accountability. While improvements to public management and financial systems are critical, it is argued that the only way to affect long-term health outcomes in developing countries—particularly for the poorest citizens—is to fundamentally reform financing and ownership structures, with an emphasis on increased use of material incentives, markets, and competition as mechanisms to allocate health resources.

Although not representing any formal statement of policy in the health sector, this cluster of studies reflected two very important developments in Bank thinking. First, there was an explicit questioning of the welfarist model of government and traditional assumptions about its role in improving health outcomes. Second, there has been a shift away from concern with the delivery of basic and primary health care to an interest in identifying and promoting major structural reform in the health sector.

The Current Policy Agenda

The *World Development Report 1993: Investing in Health* looked explicitly at the role of government and the market in health and examines the most appropriate ownership and financing arrangements to address the linked goals of improving health outcomes, reaching the poorest, and containing costs. The report stressed a three-pronged approach to achieve these goals. First, governments should foster an environment that enables households to improve health. Second, government health spending should be made more effective by reducing expenditures on the less cost-effective interventions and expanding basic public health programs and essential clinical services. Third, diversity and competition in the provision of health services and insurance should be promoted through, *inter alia*, encouraging social or private insurance for clinical services outside the essential package and by promoting competition among suppliers.

The emphasis on achieving the optimal mix of public and private financing and delivery of health services is also a theme pursued in a recent paper by Musgrove (1996). The paper classifies health care activities into three domains—*public goods, low-cost private interventions,* and *high-cost private goods*. These domains are constructed by classifying health-related activities according to their ability to generate externalities and their cost. Musgrove argues that each of these domains is subject to market failure, and each domain generates a distinct reason for the state to intervene in the market for care. In the first domain, government should finance public goods and health services with substantial externalities. In this domain, the issue of market failure is independent of costs. The second and third domains are subject to market failure only in services that are costly enough to be financed by insurance; poverty, or the inability to buy even low-cost services, is a distinct reason for public intervention. For example, in the second domain, government should regulate private health insurance or finance insurance publicly to ensure efficient and equitable access to services. In the third domain, the government should subsidize the poor by financing some minimum level of care, either directly or by financing private providers.

Nevertheless, identifying positive areas for government action does not constitute clarification of the public role in the health sector. To respond to this challenge, Musgrove developed a checklist of what government should and should not do in health. The prohibitions include: using the tax system or any system of public fees to force the poor to subsidize health care for the rich; tying public finance to public provision; and paying for health care through fee-for-service, especially when financing private providers, without other mechanisms to control expenditures. The encouraged government actions include: regulating private activity when providing information is not enough; delivering services when it is not possible to finance private providers equitably; stimulating competition in the provision of health care; and using regulation, mandates, training, and other interventions to help the private sector to function better.

The debate about the proper role for government, quasi-markets, and the private sector in health has become the basis for a new focus in Bank policy dialogue and lending for health sector reform. The agenda is closely linked to larger issues of fiscal decentralization, privatization, and improvement in the effectiveness of public sector management. This focus has increased emphasis within the Bank on economic and financial analysis in the identification of priorities for health sector reform and in selecting cost-effective health interventions. These are important developments. What is less clear is if support is being given to borrowing countries to evaluate complex policy choices and carry out major policy reforms.

Lending

Bank activities in the health sector grew rapidly after the initial policy commitment. It is useful to consider the evolution of lending in three phases. During the first period, from 1970 to 1980, the Bank approved twenty-two population projects valued at US$422 million and two nutrition projects valued at US$35 million; in 1980 it initiated its first health project in Indonesia.[12] These projects primarily focused on the development of the facilities and skills required to implement large-scale family planning programs managed by the government. As might be expected of the first efforts in a new sector, the projects had mixed results—about 59 percent of the population projects were rated as satisfactory in OED audits.

The Bank's HNP portfolio continued to grow from 1980 through 1987. From 1981 to 1987 the Bank approved sixteen population projects, twenty-six health projects, and three stand-alone nutrition projects. Total commitments in HNP grew from about US$500 million in the first decade of experience to about US$1 billion from 1981 to 1987. The performance of the population projects improved during this period, with average performance ratings of 75 percent satisfactory. Slightly more than half (sixteen of twenty-seven) of the health projects approved during this period have been completed. Figure 4.1 displays the performance ratings for all HNP projects by year of approval through fiscal 1985 compared with all projects and programs in education. (The volatility of the results is a function of the overall number of completed projects in each year.) Overall, 63 percent of completed HNP projects received satisfactory ratings, compared with 81 percent of the education projects and 73 percent of all human resources projects.

---

12. These figures are based on project classifications recorded in the MIS. As will be discussed in the second stage of the study, classification of projects as population-, health-, or nutrition-related is somewhat arbitrary, since most population projects include substantial investments in health infrastructure, and most health projects include efforts to strengthen family planning services (see World Bank 1991b, and *HNP Annual Sector Reviews* for fiscal 1988, fiscal 1990, and fiscal 1991 for more detailed discussions).

Figure 4.1: HNP Project Performance Ratings Compared with All Projects and Education Projects, by Year of Approval

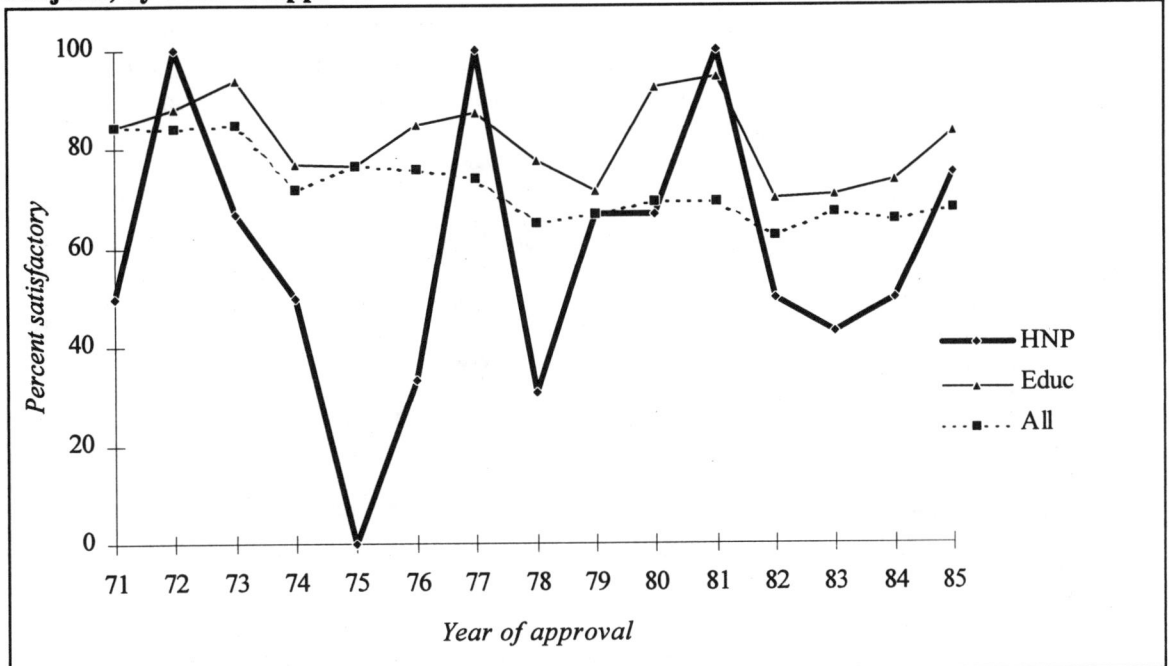

Note: This graph is based on an average of three projects annually from 1970 to 1982 (compared with twelve yearly in education). The one project in approval year 1975 was rated as unsatisfactory.

The reorganization of the Bank in 1987 and the later intensification of the Bank's commitment to HNP brought about by Mr. Conable's 1989 decision to double HNP lending resulted in rapid increases in the pace and volume of lending. This pace continues today and is reflected in figure 4.2. Since 1988 the Bank has approved ninety health projects, thirty-three population projects, and nine nutrition-related projects, representing a total loan commitment of US$1.6 billion. Projects approved since 1987 are considerably larger in scope and complexity than the programs implemented in the first fifteen years of lending in the sector. The current phase of lending demonstrates an increasing concern with major sectoral reform and efforts to address emerging health conditions, particularly the rapid increase in the prevalence of HIV infection. Project design has also become increasingly diversified. There is significant experimentation with the use of social funds and integration of health concerns into larger poverty alleviation efforts, particularly in the Latin America and Caribbean region.

Figure 4.2: Evolution of HNP Lending, by Period

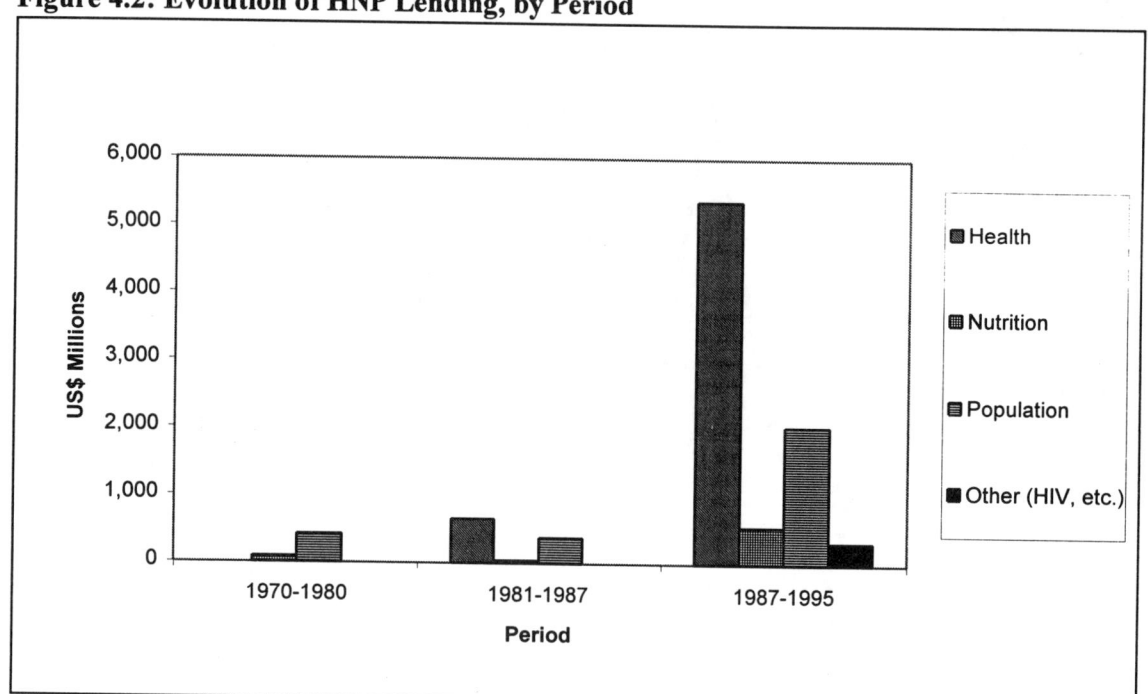

Regional Distribution

Table 4.1 provides a breakdown of all HNP lending activities from fiscal 1970 through the completion of fiscal 1996.[13] The table makes it clear that lending for health outweighs total lending for population in both total number of projects and total volume and is more evenly spread across regions, although there is a noticeable concentration in Africa and East Asia. The high volume in East Asia reflects the greater number and large size of individual loans to China. Latin America, led by Brazil (the second highest borrower in volume) is also very active in the health sector. The volume of population lending is clearly greatest in India and other countries of South Asia, although Africa is also active in the sector. Nutrition is a much less active area for stand-alone lending, although many health projects include substantial efforts to strengthen nutrition education and micronutrient supplementation. Moreover, the table does not include projects that focus on issues of food security and distribution. Overall, the Bank has committed about US$10 billion for health, population, and nutrition activities worldwide.

---

13. The data presented are based on information from the MIS, and subsectoral characterization of a project is based on data provided by operational units. In many cases, the assignment of a project to one or another category can be quite arbitrary—for example, some units might classify a "family health" project as a population project; others might classify it as a health project. We maintain the MIS classifications in this presentation, pending the possible development of a more refined typology for project classification during Phase II of the study.

Table 4.1: Regional Distribution of HNP Lending, by Subsector, Fiscal 1970–95

Area	Health	Population	Nutrition	Other	All sectors
Africa					
Number	48	18	2	7	75
Volume	1,181	476	40	140	1,836
East Asia					
Number	19	12	2	0	33
Volume	1,182	380	46.4	0	1,608
Eastern Europe and Central Asia					
Number	8	0	0	0	8
Volume	666	0	0	0	666
Latin America					
Number	26	13	5	1	45
Volume	1,630	311	193	200	2,154
Middle East and North Africa					
Number	13	6	2	2	23
Volume	481	102	12	167	761
South Asia					
Number	10	17	4	0	31
Volume	976	1,569	390	0	2,934
All regions	124	66	14	10	215
Total volume	6,115	2,837	681	326	9,959

Source: Author's calcluations based on OPRMIS data.

Distribution by Social Setting and Family Planning Program Effort

Table 4.2 shows the distribution of HNP lending by social setting, an indicator fashioned from measures of income, educational attainment, literacy, and urbanization (see Mauldin and Ross 1991, for details). Each group received a score on the most recently collected FPPI (ranked from strong to very weak/none), which serves as a proxy for the programmatic context in which a Bank project was or will be implemented. The two indicators together provide a picture of the distribution of HNP lending by social environment and family planning program performance. The latter can also be interpreted as an indicator of the performance of the health sector in basic care. Overall, the number of projects is evenly spread by social setting. About 43 percent of all projects are committed in countries classified as high or upper-middle in social setting and about 57 percent in areas with lower-middle and low social settings. It can be seen that 42 percent of HNP projects take place in settings with weak or very weak programs, 29 percent in settings with medium scores on family planning performance, and 29 percent in settings with strong programs.

Table 4.2: Number of HNP Projects in All Sectors, by Social Setting and Family Planning Program Effort Score

| Social setting | Family planning program effort score, 1990 | | | | Total | |
	Strong	Medium	Weak	Very weak/none	Number	Percentage
High	4	17	14	0	35	18.3
Upper-middle	28	17	3	0	48	25.1
Lower-middle	19	20	25	2	66	34.6
Low	5	1	29	7	42	22.0
Total	56	55	71	9	191	
Percentage	29.3	28.8	37.2	4.7		100.0

Source: Author's calculations based on OPRMIS data and W.P. Mauldin and J.A. Ross, 1991, "Family Planning Programs: Efforts and Results, 1982-1989," *Studies in Family Planning* 22(6):350-67.

Continued rapid—even explosive—growth in HNP lending is planned. The pipeline for the next four years contains ninety-two projects, and projected lending is over $7 billion—equivalent to 75 percent of all past lending. This absolute growth is reflected in the increased importance of HNP lending in overall Bank lending. HNP lending is expected to amount to 8.7 percent of total lending between fiscal 1995 and fiscal 1997—up from 5.5 percent in fiscal 1992–94 and 1.5 percent in fiscal 1986–88. The Bank is currently the largest source of international finance for the development and reform of health systems.

Reviews of HNP Work

OED Experience

OED has conducted twenty-four audits in HNP. These examinations covered eighteen population projects; fourteen of these were closed by fiscal 1984, and the most recent was closed in fiscal 1988. Four health projects, two in Malawi and two in Indonesia, were more recently audited; one nutrition project (in Colombia) was audited and one (the Tamil Nadu Integrated Nutrition Project) was subject to impact evaluation. OED has reviewed thirty-six project completion reports (PCRs) in the sector, yielding a total portfolio of sixty project evaluations (see Annex for details). Most of the early audits have little direct bearing on current health lending; they concern single-purpose family planning programs and reflect experience before the Bank's full involvement in the health sector. The completed audits have employed standard OED audit methodology. At this point, the number of active projects outnumbers the completed projects by 3 to 1, and the number of active projects outnumbers those audited by more than 10 to 1. There is clearly room for a more deliberate effort to learn from experience in this sector.

Lessons from PCRs/ICRs and PARs

A review of PCRs and PARs conducted for this paper found a number of common themes and lessons from completed projects. Although two-thirds of the projects were rated as satisfactory, a substantial majority concluded that project design had been too complex, undermining implementation and effectiveness (see Annex 2). The percentage of projects citing this problem does not vary significantly over time, indicating either that task managers have not absorbed this lesson or that incentives within the Bank continue to encourage the design of excessively complex projects. It may also indicate a lack of a clear *a priori* definition as to what constitutes project complexity. Second, a majority also cited insufficient or inadequate supervision as undermining project implementation, particularly for projects involving significant institutional reform or rural outreach. Lack of sector specialists in Resident Missions was periodic concern, particularly for sector reform programs. A few PCRs report that implementation improved when the task manager was relocated to a Resident Mission. A significant number specifically stated in the "lessons" section that current Bank arrangements for supervision were inappropriate for HNP projects.

Although nearly all completed projects include capacity building or institutional development objectives, these components experience the most difficulty and have the poorest implementation records. Problems with "software" components are noted throughout the completed portfolio and in other reviews of HNP projects. Inadequate analysis of institutional arrangements and incentives during project design and appraisal, along with inadequate supervision, were the most commonly cited reasons. Also in keeping with general Bank experience, a majority of PCRs emphasize the contribution of borrower ownership and commitment to project success, often noting that projects failed to achieve adequate ownership. Recent projects seem to indicate an increased awareness of the importance of "ownership" by Bank task teams, but even projects initiated within the past six years report problems or even cancellation because of low ownership.

Insufficient flexibility in design and implementation constrain achievement of objectives in about one-third of completed Bank projects. Several PCR report that no significant changes in design or implementation arrangements were made even in the face of highly critical supervision reports or mid-term evaluations. Conversely, a number of projects record substantial improvements in implementation following major restructuring, often resulting from negative evaluations. Finally, a large and disturbing majority report that monitoring and evaluation is either inadequate or nonexistent, making it impossible to conclude if the projects' goals are achieved. Blame for this situation was shared between Bank staff and borrower officials, usually due to a lack of interest and follow through. Most striking was that several "pilot" projects purporting to demonstrate the efficacy of a reform or new delivery system collected no evaluation data and therefore could not demonstrate whether the approach was effective.

External Reviews

Although OED has not yet conducted a major study of the effectiveness or insights gained in the Bank's work in the HNP sector, the topic has received considerable attention in a series of external and internal reviews. These studies provide an interesting overview of the questions that have concerned those responsible for the development and management of the HNP work and closely related aspects of the Bank's work in the social sectors. We provide a detailed synopsis of these studies to indicate the kinds of issues that have been addressed through assessment of the Bank's experience and to provide a basis for identifying methodological lessons and gaps in topical coverage.

Two major external reviews of Bank performance in population were commissioned. The Berelson Report (published internally in 1977) urged the Bank to focus its lending on support to large-scale family planning programs among demographically significant borrowers. The second review was completed during the reorganization of the Bank in 1987 (Simmons and Maru 1987).

The Berelson Report (1976)

Five years after the Bank began lending for population projects, an external advisory panel of population experts, led by Bernard Berelson, then President of the Population Council, was asked to provide counsel on how the World Bank could best assist member countries to lower their levels of fertility. The mandate for this major review was broad: to examine the Bank's strategies, policies, and programs, taking into consideration the Bank's role in the international community; its overall analytic and programming capacities; the strengths and weaknesses of the traditional project approach; and the political, socioeconomic, and operational conditions in developing countries. In the course of its work, the panel reviewed Bank documents; interviewed staff members working in population and other sectors, in operations and research, and in regional and country offices; and held discussions with other donors. It reviewed and appraised five of the eleven population projects, four with field visits. The panel drew on accepted views of the determinants of fertility decline in making its evaluation.

In the report to the Board, the panel organized its findings and recommendations into three major subject areas. In reviewing the first area, "The Bank's Population Policy within Development," the panel made clear its basic assumption that the Bank could equal or surpass its current achievements in bringing about fertility declines by influencing the demand for family planning through support for supply of the needed services. In the panel's view, the Bank, as the foremost general development agency, had the potential to make a major contribution in the field of population, but it had failed to utilize its comparative advantage. The panel recommended that the Bank launch an effort to realize this advantage through lending in sectors that were known to contribute to fertility decline, statements of policy by Bank leaders, policy dialogue with member countries; by incorporating population in economic reports; and by directing research toward identifying the links between population and development and making these links more relevant to operations.

The panel was less than enthusiastic about the record of "The Bank's Population Projects," the second area of the report. It found that Bank projects spent too much for staff to prepare and supervise projects and too little for the actual work of the project; and that the Bank was insufficiently flexible in design, overly ambitious in demographic objectives, and of marginal significance in the context of overall donor assistance. Yet the Berelson Report recommended continued lending, recognizing that the Bank's lending legitimated population as an area of development importance and that its support for "hardware" fulfilled a need that had not been addressed by other donors. It also acknowledged the constraints inherent in loans. The panel argued for Bank consideration of population lending focused on "key" countries. Such countries would be identified by population size, acceptance of population and family planning policies, and degree of socioeconomic advancement. It also recommended overt lending for health in programs that included family planning, arguing that the insistence on demographic targets as criteria for lending resulted in lost opportunities for broad-based health programs with likely demographic consequences. It further recommended the incorporation of family planning into other sector lending, particularly the Bank's rural development projects.

The panel found both attitudinal and organizational barriers to effective population work in its analysis of "The Bank's Population Management," the last area of its report. It proposed more training, more coordination with other population agencies, and, above all, better relationships within the Bank—first between population operations and population research, and then between the population units and the country program departments. It also recommended the appointment of a senior official to oversee these activities to ensure that population was fully incorporated into Bank activities.

Two years after publication of the first Berelson Report, two of its authors were invited to review the Bank's progress in implementing its recommendations. On the whole, they found commendable progress. On the integration of family planning into projects in other sectors, they reversed their previous recommendation, finding that it was difficult to achieve, costly in personnel, and possibly counterproductive. Instead they recommended "simultaneity" of population projects and other social sector operations.

Simmons and Maru (1988)

This second major review of the Bank's work in population was commissioned by the HNP Department in 1985 and was undertaken by two external consultants under the general direction of the Bank's senior population adviser. It was the third of three subsectoral reviews to examine performance following the integration of HNP activities in 1980. Implementation of the recommendations of this review was never monitored—partly because the report was overtaken by the 1987 reorganization and partly because HNP management never officially endorsed the review's findings. The reviewers' mandate was confined to evaluation of lending and sector activities (sector reports and research and policy dialogue), with reference to Bank organization and procedures only as they related to project performance. Consideration of staffing and skill issues was not part of the terms of reference. The team performed its evaluation through discussions with staff working in the population area, field visits, and a review of Bank documents. The team based its evaluation on a comparison of Bank performance with a theoretical framework of the factors that lead to successful population activities rather than a detailed analysis of individual projects.

The review rated overall performance as "commendable." It found that policy dialogue linking population issues with other aspects of development "perhaps the single most effective element in the Bank's work on population." The HNP Department had devoted considerable resources to sector work since its establishment in 1980, but for countries with mature programs the report recommended that sector work move from broad sectoral reviews to in-depth analysis of selected policy or program effectiveness issues, the role of NGOs, and community perspectives. Like the Berelson Report, this review also recommended a more operational focus for Bank population research.

Project performance received a mixed review in the report. The increased volume of lending, greater number of projects, and wider geographic coverage following the establishment of the HNP Department were recognized. At the same time, the reviewers found that there had been a concentration on "key" countries, and that this was useful. The team warned that the association of the Bank's population programs with health lending and the resulting reliance on generally weak ministries of health constrained population programs, and it recommended diversification to other ministries. Commenting on the heavy support for civil works and other hardware components, which averaged about 50 percent of project costs, the team recognized the importance and appropriateness of the Bank's role, given the availability of grant support for "soft" components and the greater willingness of governments to borrow for "hard" components. Nevertheless, it warned against the tendency for supervision of this component to dominate other elements of the programs. In general, the team argued for smaller, less complex projects. It advocated better design in institutional development components, more attention to delivering services at the periphery, greater involvement of NGOs, better IEC, and more effective evaluation of projects. Consideration of the use of specialists in the resident missions to provide ongoing technical assistance was also recommended.

Internal Reviews

Population and the World Bank: Implications from Eight Case Studies (OED 1992)

OED's study of the Bank's population work in eight countries is the only evaluation based on detailed analysis of country experience. To prepare the eight case studies, independent, recognized population policy experts were asked to review documents that described both lending and nonlending activities in the Bank's HNP portfolio for each country. In addition, the consultants visited each country to interview representatives of government, other donor agencies, and NGOs active in the field. The countries examined provide a cross-section of Bank involvement: Brazil, Mexico, and Colombia, where Bank population activities were minimal; Senegal, where the Bank's efforts concentrated on helping the government to develop a population policy rather than extending family planning services; Indonesia and India, where the Bank largely provided financial support for the countries' own national objectives and programs; and Bangladesh and Kenya, where the Bank played a more active role. Some 80 percent of the Bank's population lending has been applied in support of programs in the last four countries.

The report's conclusions strongly endorse calls for more emphasis in the Bank's population work on programs to influence demand through interventions that produce the conditions for fertility decline. The report confirms that fertility decline can be initiated by programs that provide contraceptive supplies, services, and associated information and that progress is more rapid when programs offer strong outreach and high-quality services designed to meet clients' perceptions of their needs. To implement such as program, first-rate field supervision, training, and motivation are required, elements that are difficult to develop in poor, rural areas. To achieve sustained fertility declines that continue until the replacement level is reached requires a variety of strategies. The Bank might have achieved more had it searched for selective interventions in development that changed the implicit benefits and costs of large families. The reorganization of the Bank was seen to offer the possibility of more effective and purposive action in this effort.

Within traditional population projects and components, there are several suggested lines of improvement. The emphasis on "hardware" was justified by the expectation that governments or other donors would provide the "software" elements, often involving recurrent costs. This expectation was shown to be overly optimistic in several of the countries studied, and a fuller array of project inputs is needed to ensure successful implementation. In addition, the tendency for a project to grow beyond the size originally planned and to take on funding of an increasing share of recurrent costs needs to be examined. The country's absorptive capacity, concerns about efficiency, and long-term sustainability must be considered. The report found that the ability of the Bank and the recipient country to assess project and program effectiveness is poor. Until project components associated with monitoring, evaluation, and research capacity are given attention, this will not change.

One of the lessons drawn from the case studies is that efforts in the population field only begin to show results after an extended period—about fifteen years. This suggests that projects should be seen as part of a broader program, and that objectives and evaluation criteria should be tailored accordingly. Nonproject activities—sector work, policy dialogue, efforts to improve organizational arrangements, more collaboration with other donors—are very important, and the Bank needs to support and reward these activities. In line with its emphasis on the importance of demand factors and the limitations imposed by absorptive capacity, the report concludes that "we find no evidence that more financial resources would have made much difference." Reorientation of activities—more nonproject activities and more lending in mutually reinforcing social sectors—would be a better use of resources.

Strengthening the Bank's Population Work in the Nineties (Sinding 1991)

Written by the Bank's second population adviser, Steven Sinding, this strategy paper drew on the conclusions of the previous reviews and a nearly completed OED study (see above) in making its recommendations. Although it was the first major look at population work in the Bank after the reorganization and the formation of country-based population and human resource divisions, it dealt almost exclusively with population and family planning issues. The paper was based on a review of levels and trends in lending, selective document review, and staff interviews.

After presenting the reasons that the Bank should continue involvement in population, Sinding concluded that there are countries where the macroeconomic consequences of population growth are sufficiently threatening to development to warrant attention to population issues. In most countries, he noted, family planning serves primarily to improve the lives of individuals, most notably their health. He then presented a conceptual framework, similar to that proposed by the Berelson Panel, but more fully developed over time, for deciding on appropriate strategies, given the degree of program effort and a country's level of socioeconomic development (their "social setting"). Sinding argued that the most critical elements for successful Bank population projects are government commitment; the strengthening of existing institutions rather than the creation of new ones; a greater involvement of the private sector and enhanced quality through training, transport, and logistics; adequate management information; and a suitable and reliable contraceptive supply. His main conclusion, however, was that it is difficult to evaluate the effectiveness of Bank population work because no coherent, sustained effort has been made to develop the necessary indicators.

Review of HNP Lending for Health (Measham 1985)

This review of the HNP Department's first five years of experience dealt with health projects and the health components of combined HNP projects. It looked at the level of effort in sector work and lending and adherence to the directions enumerated in the 1980 *Health Policy Paper*. The paper was based on a detailed content analysis of documentation of ongoing sector work and lending operations (at various stages of development). The study did not include explicit objective indicators of performance, but instead relied on the author's assessment of the relevance and potential effectiveness of these operations.

The review endorsed the attention given to sector work that preceded HNP projects in all but a handful of countries with projects under supervision or in preparation. Sector work was found to have led to increased staff effectiveness, greater Bank credibility with borrowing countries and with the Bank's country program departments, changes in policy in several countries, and increased lending. The majority of sector reports were broad reviews, appropriate to a new area of lending. While the findings concerning sector work confirmed the statements in the 1980 document about the importance of primary health care and the imbalance in health expenditure allocations in most countries, they also identified several significant areas not treated in the policy paper that are important to an understanding of country conditions and the selection of appropriate interventions. Chief among these were of health costs and financing, "an area of strength in HNP sector work" and an area of major comparative advantage for the Bank; the hospital sector, which consumes most health resources and must be understood in order to achieve some reallocation; urban health problems; chronic diseases; and health support systems.

The major recommendations included increased sector work that concentrates on in-depth analysis of one issue and more sharply focused "second-generation" projects. Greater national involvement in sector work should be sought, and HNP should seek greater participation in public investment reviews. The report urged that projects develop cost-effective models of health care delivery, with greater attention to NGOs and the private sector. There should be more effort to incorporate methods to evaluate projects; employment of process indicators as quantifiable targets was seen as generally inappropriate. The report advocated increased understanding of service delivery at the periphery—to groups underserved by reason of geography or poverty. It recommended that studies of demand and utilization patterns be included in sector work and project preparation to aid in effective design. No documentation of the degree of adoption of this recommendation is available.

Nutrition Review (Skolnik and others 1987)

This review largely focused on operational experience and brought together the lessons of the four free-standing nutrition projects approved since 1975; to a lesser extent, it included nutrition components in HNP projects and other sector projects. Skolnik and others found that the projects had been too complex and had tried to deal with too many of the causes of malnutrition. They were nonetheless largely successful in bringing about nutritional improvement in environments that had experienced little increase in income. Lack of a single responsible entity within a country hampered the management of nutrition projects; attention must be given to institution building. Targeting had been shown to be a practical and cost-effective way of providing food and services with maximum impact, and the projects were important in attracting policy attention and resources to the problems of malnutrition.

The report recommended greater attention to nutrition in population and health projects, given the potential of nutrition projects and components to contribute to primary health care and family planning programs. It suggested three kinds of projects, defined by content: (a) nutrition projects to improve infant and child health; (b) nutrition to improve human capital formation and labor productivity through increased availability of food for a household; and (c) control of the major micronutrient deficiency diseases. While recommendations (a) and (c) fell within the purview of the HNP Department, expertise in the area of recommendation (b) involved food subsidy programs, institutional feeding projects, and improved efficiency in the food marketing system and would have to be developed slowly. The report identified Bank research as having played an important role in advancing the understanding of costs and cost-effectiveness in nutrition programs.

Reaching the Poor: HNP Performance at the Periphery (Heaver 1988)

Although not conducted as a formal review, this working paper focused on the ability of HNP projects to make a difference "on the ground." The author compared the characteristics of client populations at the periphery with the standard government health care system and found them mismatched. He argued that HNP service delivery systems must be adapted to local conditions to maximize service utilization.

This review, again based on content analysis of documents for ongoing projects, indicated that the vast majority of projects had included extension of coverage and/or the quality of HNP services to poorly served populations among their objectives. No less than 69 percent of projects used community health workers to deliver services and provide education. IEC was included in 85 percent of the projects, and over half involved the mobilization of community support groups to encourage the acceptance of IEC or health services. Nevertheless, the report found that the Bank's knowledge of the determinants of the behavior of both clients and service providers was too scanty to ensure that outreach systems and IEC services were designed to accommodate the needs and circumstances of the client population. The review also found that the Bank had not done enough to target project-financed services to priority clients, particularly the most disadvantaged groups at the periphery.

Heaver made detailed recommendations for sector work, lending, policy, and research to remedy this lack—including greater efforts to understand and accommodate the clients' perspective in the design of outreach and IEC components; increased use of alternative modes of delivery such as NGOs and the private sector; more comprehensive identification of client groups; and the development of appropriate output and process targets. He points out that while in the private sector a firm that fails to be responsive to its customers goes bankrupt, a public health care clinic that fails to meet its clients' needs can survive indefinitely with low levels of utilization.

Analyses of Human Development: Supporting Human Development—Progress and Challenges

The Population and Human Resources Department prepared this review of Bank experience in the human development sector—defined as education, training, health, nutrition, population, employment, and the socioeconomic role of women—at the request of the Board. The paper described the situation before the Bank's 1987 reorganization in broad terms—the expanding rationales for involvement, the increase in lending, and the entry into new areas based on research and sector work, allied with increased flexibility in lending instruments.

Nevertheless, the paper came to the overall conclusion that "the early lending focus on the implementation of specific interventions often resulted in weak links with country assistance strategies," especially in the health, nutrition, and population sectors, which were centralized in the Operational Policy Staff (OPS) vice-presidency. The organizational separation of units on education, HNP, and WID virtually precluded the formulation of coordinated human development strategies as an integral part of country assistance strategies. This hampered the ability of the Bank to deal effectively with the social impact of adjustment programs, and to design coherent strategies for poverty alleviation and technological capacity-building.

The reorganization increased the visibility and centrality of human development in the country dialogue and provided a framework for the exploitation of the complementarities and synergies among the different elements. It did this by integrating operational responsibility for human development programs in a single division in each country department, supported by a division in each regional technical department, and by concentrating research and policy work in a central department. Thus, it created the conditions for rapid evolution of the Bank's role in the sector through integrating human development in country assistance strategies; expanding the lending program; broadening lending objectives; increasing the use of diverse lending instruments; strengthening quality and operational focus of research and policy analyses on human development, and collaborating with a broad range of partners in program design and implementation.

Lessons learned in the sector reinforce the importance of the conditions detailed above. Most important, a well-designed policy and institutional framework can provide wide access to basic human development services, even in low-income countries. Without such a framework, increases in GNP alone often do not improve the lives of the poor. Experience has shown that project-specific investment loans do not always yield desired policy change, and that sectoral reform must be approached as more than the sum of individual investments. Bank support has been most effective when based on sector-wide programs of reform and development; in-depth analysis of sectoral issues; building national capacity for program design and implementation; continuous attention to implementation, and systematic monitoring of outcomes.

Reviewers' Comments on the Bank's Measurement of Project Performance

In addition to the broad studies of population programs, the Bank also commissioned a study of the use of targets and indicators in population projects, a relevant topic given the emphasis on the problems of weak monitoring and evaluation detailed in studies of Bank experience. The most comprehensive look at targets and indicators was undertaken by Baldwin (1992), who brought the benefit of his years of experience in operations to the evaluation of the Bank's performance in setting targets in population projects and its measurement of impact. He first distinguished between input and output measures and then subdivided each category. Input indicators include measures of project implementation and process; output indicators include measures of performance and ultimate impact. While the two input variables are both project-related, Baldwin argued that measurement of output variables is generally only feasible at the program level. At the project level, measurement of outputs can only be done where it is possible to separate the project catchment area from the national program. He is therefore critical of suggestions (for example, Simmons and Maru 1988; World Bank 1991b) that the Bank be more rigorous in establishing output targets and indicators for projects. He found these statements generally platitudinous and not "actionable." His recommendation was to pay attention to input indicators at the project level, and to output indicators at the program level. (In this respect, he noted that the OED study ends by recommending output indicators that measure progress toward sectoral goals.) Baldwin was also more in favor of using output indicators than targets—looking for trends in the right direction rather than deciding if a specific goal has been achieved. Monitoring trends involves comparison: to a target, if one has been set, or to a country's past performance, or to the performance of other countries.

In reviewing the Bank instruments used to evaluate projects, Baldwin found the most to praise in the staff appraisal reports (SARs) of follow-on projects. He noted that they are a rich source of information on past program and project performance. He was most critical of OED performance audit reports (PARs). Of the Malaysia audit report, Baldwin wrote that "OED reviews and judgments deserve a high place on the agenda of professional discussion about how to assess the worthwhileness of Bank population projects—but no more. They do not deserve any extraordinary deference simply because they represent the Bank's 'judgment of last resort' in a sequence of formal procedures. Whether or not PARs add significantly to the data and insights of PCRs is a separate, important issue. My own view, based solely on my reading of the 18 population PARs done to date, is that the cost of conducting PARs far outweighs their benefits." He goes on to recommend devoting these resources to operational research on specific topics and to general reviews of national programs.

In detailing the distinction between indicators appropriate to projects and those appropriate to programs and in his recommendation that output indicators emphasize program achievements, Baldwin echoes the broad conclusions of the Berelson Panel. They found: "As for the more specific targets, in fertility rates of one kind or another, they seem ill-attached to the project, unrealistic, fitted to too short a time period, and in any case difficult perhaps impossible of reliable measurement and attribution to the project in the current state of the art" (Berelson and Freedman 1976, p. 39).

Simmons and Maru (1988) were more critical of Bank performance in this area. They quoted with approval an OED audit criticizing the lack of a specific framework in the project under review "on the basis of which causal relationships can be established between the project's stated objectives on the one hand and project activities on the other. As a result, there is no hard 'causal' evidence as to the extent that 'micro' project activities contributed to the 'macro' project activities." Beyond recommending that Bank staff familiarize themselves with UN papers that outline alternative approaches, however, the report made no specific recommendations.

Sinding (1991) was similarly critical. Rather than accepting that it has been difficult to assess the effectiveness of Bank projects to reduce fertility because of the problems of distinguishing among project, program, and other development interventions, he argued that: "It is not easy to attribute fertility decline, or even increased contraceptive prevalence, to a single project, but if the project represents a substantial element of a country's population program, it is not unreasonable to infer that a substantial share of any observed change is attributable to the project." The question of time lags was not raised. Sinding was also rather general in his recommendation that the Bank begin to think more consistently about population objectives, calling for explicit population objectives, consistent with those of the country in question; careful provision for data collection and analysis, through service statistics and periodic surveys, for example; and inclusion of an impact evaluation component in projects to assure greater attention to basic objectives.

The only major review of health lending (Measham 1986), however, contains recommendations that are more in line with those of the later Baldwin report. Measham commented that "verifying the achievement of mortality targets is difficult, especially in the case of maternal mortality. But even for infant and child mortality, which are in principle easier to measure reliably, few countries have the capability to mount area-specific baseline and post-project surveys of these parameters. Except in the exceptional case where the capability clearly exists, it seems preferable not to rely on quantified mortality reductions to measure project impact" (pp. 27–28). Measham recommended, as did Baldwin, the use of process or activity data that can be used to estimate impact where other parameters are known—use of immunization coverage where disease-specific mortality rates are known, for example. Other important indicators of health care coverage—for example, antenatal care—are less easily translated into outcome measures. Nevertheless, they represent the most practical set of indicators for use as the basis of judgments about the success of health projects in improving health status.

In sum, reviewers who provided concrete advice on the use of targets and indicators in Bank projects were most likely to recommend careful accounting of Bank project funds through measurement of input indicators, with output indicators measured at the national or program level through surveys or data systems independent of service statistics.

Key Performance Indicators for HNP

Review of a random sample of completion and audit reports for complete HNP projects reveals gaps in monitoring and evaluation systems. As summarized in Table 4.3, problems include from the failure to design an adequate monitoring system, a tendency for M&E systems to focus on inputs rather than outputs or impacts, unreliable reports from the systems that are established, and failure to specify procedures to enhance the use of monitoring information in making decisions at either the project or sectoral context.

Work to strengthen monitoring and evaluation in the HNP sector received renewed attention following the production of the Wapenhans report. To assist Bank staff to identify and use indicators to improve the monitoring and evaluation of projects the Health, Nutrition, and Population Department prepared an analysis of HNP indicators in 1995 (World Bank 1995d). The paper recommends indicators to assess project inputs, processes, outputs, and outcomes. The paper notes that because of the diversity of project objectives and the benefits of country specificity, it is not possible to identify a single set of indicators that can be used across all HNP lending operations. Rather, the paper presents a list of indicators to measure service output of a range of specific intervention categories and suggests that project preparation teams select from this list. The list of also includes indicators of the organizational and managerial characteristics of particular program structures, but does not propose criteria for evaluating health care system performance.

The paper recommends that careful specification of project objectives and planning for collection of baseline data during preparation and appraisal would facilitate evaluation of program impact. The paper does not report on past experience with the implementation of these recommendations, but notes that capacity for monitoring and evaluation among borrower agencies is often limited. The paper further notes that borrower and stakeholder participation in the specificational objectives can be a useful device for strengthening ownership and understanding of project objectives. The paper does not address questions concerning how to evaluate progress in strengthening sectoral capacity as a whole, the specification of indicators of institutional change within the sector, nor the evaluation of multi-intervention programs.

Table 4.3: Comments on Monitoring and Evaluation from PCR/ICR and/or Audit Reports

Country, Project Title, Loan/Credit Number	
Burkina Faso: Health Services Development Project (1986-1994) C1607	"...the lack of a monitoring system and of monitorable indicators makes it particularly difficult to measure project impact." (p. iv)
Colombia: Health Services Integration Project (1985-1993) L2611	Borrower's comments: "The program design did not make any provision for the use of specific instruments, variables, or indicators to be used in monitoring and evaluating the project and assessing its benefits to the Government, in particular to the health sector. Only in the last stage, when actions were focusing on Law 10 and its implementation, were a few M&E instruments available, both for the various project processes and for the expected results." (p. 14-15) "The Bank's system of project monitoring and control was not apparent." General recommendations for other projects: "The Bank should endeavor to systematize its monitoring and supervision procedures and to ensure their constant application." (p. 17-18)
The Gambia: National Health Development Project (1987-1995) C1760	"Key indicators for project operation were neither contained in the SAR or the DCA, nor were they elaborated during project life." (p. 18) Lessons learned: "Efforts should be made to compile reliable baseline data in order to set realistic and clear targets and to define easily measurable indicators." (p. 10)
India: Fourth Population Project (1985-1994) C1623	"A series of surveys and research reports, including baseline, mid-term, and end-of-project surveys were carried out with project support....There has been little appreciation of the potential usefulness of research results in the India population projects. The attitude of managers in West Bengal was different; many improvements in program implementation can be traced directly to research findings." (p. 6)
Indonesia: Provincial Health Project (1983-1989) L2235	"The evaluation data presented as of the Closing Date is <u>unreliable</u> as it is under-reported and possibly inconsistent. Although data was collected for the Monitoring and Evaluation Indicators established for the project, they have not been systematically collected or analyzed, given the delays in the commissioning of the facilities, and, consequently, delays in acquiring data. Further some of the indicators established during the appraisal are also unrealistic. Borrower performance: "The lack of full time staff has resulted in reporting, recording and monitoring and evaluation systems established that are less than adequate." (p. 8) "Impact, coverage and health status indicators were developed for monitoring and evaluation of the project, but the system is not yet fully operational due to delays in the commissioning of the facilities, and inconsistent reporting from the field." (p. 5) "In both projects [this one and the Nutrition and Community Health project] most quantifiable and monitorable indicators are for input, very few, such as number of persons trained, for output, and basically none for monitoring or evaluating effects." (Audit, p. 14)
Indonesia: Second Nutrition and Community Health Project (1985-1991) L2636	"Although no quantitative target [sic] were set against which to assess effects, the project did a study of Posyandu utilization which was also useful for this audit." (Audit, p. 14) "In both projects [this one and the Provincial health project] most quantifiable and monitorable indicators are for input, very few, such as number of persons trained, for output, and basically none for monitoring or evaluating effects." (Audit, p. 14)
Malawi: Second Family Health Project (1987-1993) C1768	"Quantifying project impact is not possible because no baseline data was available to compare with; the lack of clearly identified monitoring indicators in the project documents also contribute to quantifying difficulties." (p. i) "It is not possible to quantify the impact of the project because no surveys were carried out before the start, or at the end, of the project. Difficulty in quantifying results can also be ascribed to the lack of clearly identified monitoring indicators in project documents, lack of institutional memory, and reports which appear to conflict with evidence in the field." (p. 6)

Table 4.3 (Continued)

Country, Project Title, Loan/Credit Number	
Mali: Health Development Project (1983-1991) C1422	"The SAR did not precisely identify what the project hoped to achieve at the village level; specifically, it did not identify measurable indicators or a process which might be monitored and modified. The monitoring, research, and evaluation component indicated nothing about an information feedback loop." (p. 9) "Belgian technicians developed planning and coordination activities for a monitoring and evaluation system: their design involved monitoring at the central level without feedback; the information collected was not immediately utilized." (p. iii)
Rwanda: Family Health Project (1986-1993) C1678	"...most of the performance indictors in the SAR were exceeded. However, it should be noted that they were not systematically monitored during project supervision and were not included in the progress reports." (p. 8)
Senegal: Rural Health Project (1982-1991) C1310	"In the end, the capacities of the Ministry were strengthened, particularly with respect to decentralized planning, personnel management and project evaluation." (p. 7) No further information provided.
Tunisia: Health and Population Project (1981-1989) L2005	"The lack of a functioning [MIS] system meant that baseline project indicators were never updated as planned and the project monitoring database was poor, making determinations of health service outreach and attainment of specific project goals difficult to measure." (p. 9) "...the impact of the project is difficult to measure as the MIS, which was supposed to monitor specific project indicators, never functioned as planned and no results are available about the project's goals of increased coverage, reduction in IMR, CBR, and morbidity." (Audit, p. 35)
Yemen, Republic of : Second Health Development Project (1988-95) C1972	"Monitoring Outcomes. Since most civil works activities were not completed until the last year of project implementation, it was difficult to measure their impact on the achievement of project objectives." (p. 7) All facilities constructed were reported to be staffed and operational. "In terms of their effectiveness as a means to expand access to PHC services, the number of patients being treated per day at the primary health care units (PHCU) varies from 2 to 20, which suggests that more people now have access to primary services. However, a survey of the catchment population found that, on average, 60 percent of the people thought that the services provided by the PHCUs were insufficient to meet their basic needs and the facilities were found to be providing about half of the services which they were expected to provide. Source: 'Project Assessment Study', March 1996. The survey is not representative of the population therefore the results are only indicative." (pp. 2-3) No monitoring and evaluation indicators mentioned in the ICR.
Zimbabwe: Family Health Project (1986-1993) L2744	A baseline survey was carried out at the start of the project, as well as a mid-term review, and end-of-project survey, and an independent district management survey in the third year. These surveys were not particularly well done, although considerable effort was put into them but many useful data were collected. The data at appraisal and PCR are not perfectly comparable because the indicators have been defined differently for the different stages.

Implications for Evaluation

Although the HNP portfolio has not been subject to intensive audit work and coverage of health projects is particularly scanty, previous reviews do provide suggestions for considerations of development effectiveness in the sector. Three themes raised throughout these reviews appear particularly noteworthy.

First, there is recognition throughout the reviews that the Bank must be concerned with the demand for HNP services as well as their supply. This was raised most explicitly as part of the effort to define the Bank's appropriate role in population policy and emerges again in OED's own evaluation of population projects. The more limited reviews of health programs fail to make an issue of demand questions, although there is evidence in the evaluation literature that these variables are important elements in choice of service provider. Much of the current thinking about the health sector and the advantages and disadvantages of alternative delivery systems, however, appears to assume that demand, particularly for the "minimum essential package of services," exists, and the question is merely how best to meet it. The increasing recognition that many public health and clinical health interventions require "behavior change" suggests that HNP activities must be more cognizant of factors that affect family health-seeking behaviors, particularly patterns influencing choice of provider. Most reviews are relatively silent on just how such demand-side variables should be accommodated in the design of delivery systems, which suggests that an ex post review of actual utilization patterns could be useful in developing guidance in this area.

One theme, most explicitly treated in the human development strategy documents, implies that both supply and demand questions are best managed at the macroeconomic level by ensuring a close fit between HNP activities and other elements of the country assistance strategy. The paper argues that the 1987 reorganization provided the opportunity to overcome many of the constraints that had been shown to limit effectiveness by encouraging greater country specificity in the design of activities. Analyses of development effectiveness could fruitfully ask how such a broad sectoral approach could be operationalized. Has the shift to country specificity produced a shift in the content, level, and form of lending instruments? What is the relationship between these shifts and the emerging consensus on the need for sector reform projects?

The tensions between the Bank's apparent focus on the provision of "hardware" through its project lending and the need at the country level for "improved software" are also repeated in several reviews. Interpreting the concept of "software" to refer to some combination of borrower decisions on what services to provide and determinations of how to provide them suggests that assessment of the Bank's performance in the provision of software will require consideration of the processes it uses to identify how decisions are made in a given country as well as its influence on the outcome of these decisions.

It is clear that the HNP field has not suffered from a lack of voices arguing for new and better methods of monitoring and evaluation. As OED's studies of monitoring and evaluation document, HNP compares well with other sectoral groups in the Bank in the incorporation of appropriate monitoring and evaluation systems in project appraisal reports. Conversely, HNP has been no more successful than others in solving the problem of building institutional capacity for monitoring and evaluation among its borrowers.

5.   Assessing Development Effectiveness in HNP

From a modest start 25 years ago, the World Bank has become the world's largest lender in the health, nutrition, and population sectors. Today, the Bank also plays a leading role as an advisor on national health policies, often advocating reforms to promote efficiency, cost-effectiveness, and attention to emerging health problems, including the HIV epidemic. In parallel, the Bank has reduced its emphasis on project lending for public family planning and basic health services and increased its support for projects aimed at sector reform, especially projects that seek to redress inter- and intrasectoral imbalances in health expenditures and change the balance between public and private roles in the sector. These shifts are occurring rapidly and in a health portfolio that is increasing in volume and complexity. Despite the rapid expansion of its lending and the breadth and depth of its analytic work in HNP, the Bank has not yet attempted a review of the effectiveness of its activities in the sector. Thus, an evaluation of the development effectiveness of the Bank's HNP activities is timely. This chapter outlines the elements of such an assessment and how it might be undertaken, drawing on the literature reviewed in earlier chapters on health and fertility transitions, previous efforts to evaluate health programs and policies, and assessments of the Bank's experience in HNP.

Lessons for Evaluation. The previous chapters suggest two major challenges for an evaluation of HNP. First, health outcomes are determined by a complex array of influences in addition to health services. The most important are income, nutritional status, education, and the quality of the environment—particularly access to safe water and sanitation. The provision of health services is but one of the variables that influence health, fertility, and nutrition outcomes. It is therefore difficult to establish clear causal links between specific health interventions and improvements in health outcomes.

Second, although there has been considerable evaluative research on specific disease interventions, the literature provides little guidance on how to assess the performance of health care systems as a whole. The behavior of individuals is the primary determinant of health status and fertility. In contrast, health programs and projects operate by altering the health care system rather than individual behaviors. Even projects targeted at specific diseases, nutritional deficiencies, and high fertility usually operate through increasing country capacity to meet these challenges through the health system.

Figure 5.1 shows two major paths through which health outcomes (fertility, mortality, nutritional status) might change. First, individual or household characteristics can affect health outcomes both directly and indirectly. People's knowledge, attitudes, and behavior can have a direct influence on health status, independent of the formal health care system. In addition, changes in individual or household characteristics can alter the demand for health goods and services, independent of any changes in the health system itself. Second, health care systems affect health outcomes directly by affecting the mix, quality, supply, and private costs of health care services, and indirectly by promoting consumer demand for health care services and by encouraging healthy behavior.

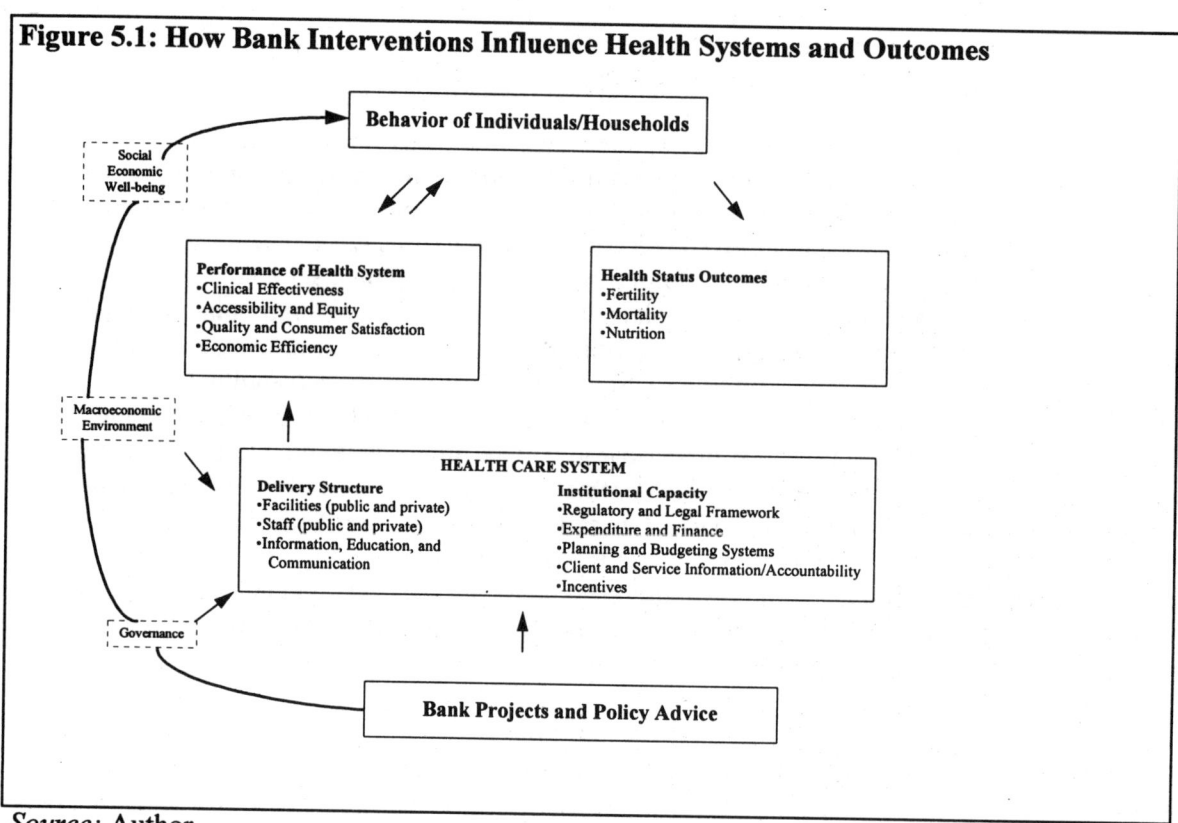

Figure 5.1: How Bank Interventions Influence Health Systems and Outcomes

Source: Author.

Figure 5.1 also shows that the structure and institutional capacity of the health care system influences the accessibility, efficiency, quality, and effectiveness of services. The quality and availability of health services (from both public and private providers) not only affect the effectiveness of treatment or prevention of disease, but also influence demand. If consumer satisfaction is low, services will not be used even if they are accessible and clinically effective.

Economics, politics and national "governance" guide health expenditures and financing arrangements which help determine system performance. Each country's health care system is shaped by the size and character of private sector providers and interests, the size and placement of voluntary agencies, and the efficiency and effectiveness of public sector management. Ongoing work in the "new institutional economics" suggests that the institutional environment influences success in providing goods of different types. Public goods, for instance, may be more effectively delivered in less hierarchical settings (Picciotto 1995). Although empirical tests of these relationships are only now being developed, governance and macroeconomic performance must be considered in assessing and comparing project performance over time and across countries.

The socioeconomic environment strongly influences household behavior. For example, changes in income, education, or access to transport and communications can alter attitudes toward specific health behaviors (e.g., breastfeeding, smoking, and diet and exercise routines) and thereby influence health outcomes even in the absence of deliberate programs. Furthermore, changes in the environment can influence changes in the demand for health goods and services independent of any change in the health care system itself. Determining the strength of these influences, relative to changes attributable to the health care system itself, is an important research question which remains unanswered in most countries.[14]

Bank policy advice and projects, therefore, can influence health outcomes through two complex pathways. First, Bank policy advice and investments could change health outcomes by improving socioeconomic well-being, increasing family income and access to food, education, and clean water. Second, policy advice and projects could influence health outcomes through strengthening the "health care system" by expanding facilities; adjusting the role of public, private, and voluntary providers; improving the skills of health providers; or through adjusting the institutions that contribute to health system performance.

There are two important implications for the evaluation of the Bank's HNP activities that follow from these interactions. First, although non-health Bank interventions clearly affect health outcomes through improved socioeconomic well-being, analyzing such links is well beyond the scope of this study (though analysis of the degree to which project selection and design recognize such links is not). Second, although improved health outcomes are the ultimate measure of Bank effectiveness, Bank health lending and policy dialogue are mediated through the health care system. Thus, an evaluation must focus primarily on how the Bank has influenced health systems through HNP lending and policy advice, taking account of both the supply and demand for health services.[15]

Three other considerations also justify concentrating on systems rather than outcomes. First, as noted in Chapter 4, the explosion in Bank lending for HNP in the past decade means that the majority of Bank HNP projects and funds are invested in ongoing projects. These projects are too important and numerous not to be assessed, but are too recent to have affected health outcomes. Second, most of this "new generation" of projects aim to improve the health care system, rather than simply expand services. Third, although an assessment of the interaction between the health care system and outcomes would be ideal, most completed HNP projects failed to collect data on project impact and thus provide no basis for linking projects to outcomes (see Table 4.3).

The remainder of this chapter is organized into four parts. First, an evaluative framework for studying health systems is outlined. Second, plans for a cross-country analysis of Bank lending throughout the HNP sector to provide an overview of current and past Bank activities in HNP are laid out. Third, a series of country sector impact studies that constitute the heart of the evaluation are described. Fourth and last, expected results and outputs are described.

---

14. Gertler and Molyneaux (1994) recently developed an analysis of Indonesia's fertility transition employing a model roughly analogous to what would be required for this level of analysis. The data available, however, did not allow an analysis of the health transition, despite Indonesia's relatively rich stock of useable data. Gathering the data to test such a model is well beyond the resources available to most studies. Moreover, such analyses are likely to confirm that health services account for only a small portion of the variance in health outcomes. Thus, they would provide little direct information on how to improve efficiency, effectiveness or quality within the bounds of the existing institutional apparatus.

15. One important dimension along which projects vary is the degree to which they specifically aim to achieve changes in health outcome. Specific disease control efforts, for instance to control malaria or HIV infections, may be expected to result in specific identifiable changes in outcome. Other projects aim to strengthen particular aspects of health system performance and may or may not anticipate changes in health outcomes. Still others aim at a mix of system improvement and disease control and prevention, suggesting that many projects cannot be assessed relative to change in health outcome.

Toward an Evaluation Framework

Although it is difficult to quantify how much a country's health care system contributes to the healthiness of its citizens, some health systems are recognizably better than others. And most observers, including the World Bank, continue to believe that improving the performance of a country's health care system is an important policy objective. Two features of national health care systems provide the major channel through which policy choices and changes in incentives influence the performance of the system. First, the structure of service delivery, that is the number and type of health facilities, the number and type of staff, and their distribution among public, private, or voluntary agencies, determines the degree to which the goods and services produced do or do not *respond to consumer demand*. Second, each system's *institutional capacity* governs the flow of resources (providers, consumers, equipment, and supplies) in and out of these facilities and their associated service outputs.[16] It is useful to consider the relevance of these two elements of the system to an analysis of how the Bank does, or might influence the performance of the system.

The health sector in most countries is not managed by any single, monolithic agency. It usually includes a number of governmental agencies, such as Ministries of Health, Ministries of Social Welfare, various levels of local administration, nongovernmental organizations, and of course, private providers and various groups representing the interests of professional or consumer groups. Efforts to improve sectoral policy, whether targeted on the implementation of a disease-specific programs or on broader issues such as reform of health financing, must recognize the complexity of the decision making environment in which they are to take place. Most Bank policy and lending activities often involve changing decisions or practices across a number of agencies. To be effective, they need to encompasses formal and informal procedures that reinforce accountability, systems for gathering and interpreting information about services and their use by consumer populations, and other "rules of the game." For example, improving access to services in outlying areas requires not only training providers in the necessary clinical skills but also adjusting the incentives that govern providers' decisions to locate in rural areas. To take another example, clinical effectiveness depends on the quality of medical education, which in turn depends on the institutional and incentive structures facing universities and secondary schools. Efforts to enhance institutional capacity in this broad sense rely heavily on detailed analysis of incentives, institutions, and on a careful political analysis of organizations and interest groups.

The demand-responsiveness of the structure of service delivery is important because, to be effective, health goods and services must be consumed. A critical issue for health policy (especially where market signals are absent) is to ensure that the production of health goods and services is consistent with the demand for them, or where there are information failures that public policy and actions stimulate demand for goods and services that can make a difference in health outcomes. In other words, analyses or suggestions on how best to organize the structure of health services must be grounded in an analysis of the basic demand conditions that health services must address.[17]

---

16. The term *institutional capacity* relates primarily to managerial practices and procedures that govern the transfer of information, finance, and staff among organizations, including planning and budgeting systems.

17. Recent analyses of the demand for health care (Alderman and Levy 1996; Shaw and Griffin 1994), show that consumers are highly responsive to the characteristics of service delivery, including the perceived quality of the

Attentiveness to demand in health care entails not only responding to demand, but changing the demand for both private and public goods.[18] To be effective, health systems therefore need to seek to alter demand through the provision of information, education, and communication efforts designed to change health-related behaviors. A review of the health goods and services that would be included in a list of health priorities for most developing countries shows that most of these interventions require significant changes in target population belief patterns and behaviors, changes induced not by clinical/medical work, but by effective communication, education and promotional efforts.

If the key levers for influencing the performance of the health system are its service delivery structure and its institutional capacity, what are appropriate ways of assessing how well a system is performing ? Four evaluative criteria are suggested:[19]

1. **Clinical/Epidemiological Effectiveness** reflects how effectively and how appropriately health care providers administer medical or preventive procedures and advice. For example, at the individual level, providing a nutritional supplement to a patient who is well nourished is clearly inappropriate and will have little biological or clinical effect. Or, at the level of a system, the provision of a chloroquine regimen in areas in which resistant strains of malaria prevail would be clinically ineffective. Determining clinical effectiveness requires a diagnosis of the underlying biological constraints to good health based on thorough analysis of available epidemiological and demographic data. As discussed in Chapter 3, clinical effectiveness is hard to measure because of the difficulties of measuring health outcomes even for a single intervention and is especially difficult for multiple interventions.

2. **Accessibility and Equity** reflect how often the population and its subgroups utilize the health system. Access can be defined in numerous ways including physical accessibility, financial affordability, realized access (utilization), or in terms of equality of health outcomes. Equity is generally defined in terms of the progressivity of the contributions (i.e., taxes, premiums, out-of-pocket payments) to finance health care or in terms of access by different population subgroups. Some access indicators can be obtained from available population data, but in general, there is no more than modest information about utilization by income class.

---

providers, the costs of services, the availability of drugs and supplies, and geographic accessibility (time and travel costs). The dimensions of perceived quality are better documented in the family planning field, where it is clear that variables such as the social distance between providers and consumers and the quality and depth of counseling influence household decisions on service use. The relevance of these variables and the need to better understand the quality of services as perceived by consumers in Bank HNP lending has been studied by Heaver (1986) who shows that 69 percent of HNP projects appraised through FY86 included objectives that could be met only through the development of client-responsive services, but lacked adequate design or implementation arrangements to encourage them.

18. Individuals might consume an inappropriate amount of health care services because of a gap between medical "need" and demand (imperfect information), because others derive benefits from their healthiness (positive externalities), because insurance markets fail (moral hazard), or because parents do not always act in their children's best interest (principal-agent problem) (Musgrove 1996).

19. These criteria and their definitions were identified by Schieber (1994) and were recently employed in a sector study in the Hashemite Kingdom of Jordan (World Bank 1996).

3.   **Quality and Consumer Satisfaction** are measured through formal standards and procedures (e.g., facility accreditation, certification and licensing procedures, etc.) and as perceived by consumers. Consumer satisfaction can be measured by surveys and by revealed preference in service utilization data (when available).

4.   **Economic Efficiency** measures how efficiently the nation mobilizes and expends resources for health care. Sectoral or external efficiency refers to the total amount spent on health care and its likely implications for health outcomes. Microeconomic or internal efficiency refers to the efficiency with which services are delivered by individual institutions to individual consumers. It has a number of dimensions, including the efficiency of the system comprising all such facilities (e.g., all health centers), and the efficiency with which different services are substituted for each other. One common method used to measure efficiency is to compare unit costs across facilities holding the level and mix of patient cases constant.

Recently, a measure of health outcome has been developed which combines clinical effectiveness and economic efficiency into a measure based on the disability adjusted life year, or DALY (WDR 1993; Bobadilla and others 1994). This measure scores the number of years and quality of life lost as a result of ill-health, using a 3 percent discount rate to compute the present value of years of life gained through mitigation or prevention of disease. The resulting estimates of the costs of specific interventions can then be used to rank interventions according to the cost at which they deliver a DALY. While an important step forward, DALYs do not allow for the inevitable geographic, institutional, and temporal variation in the cost-effectiveness of various medical interventions. The effectiveness of treatments might vary, for instance, by facility, by the level of subnational government administering the system, or by whether the treatment is provided by the public or private sector. Cost-effectiveness also depends on the preferences and behavior of patients and consumers, including the biological and social characteristics of the target group for any intervention, as well as on temporal changes in demand for services. In other words, at present there exists no single measure for the overall performance of health care systems; evaluations must pursue all four evaluative criteria mentioned in the last paragraph.

In past decades policymakers in developing countries generally emphasized the first and second criteria, equal access and clinical effectiveness, over the third and fourth criteria, consumer satisfaction and economic efficiency. As in other sectors of the economy, central planning was used to allocate capital investment in the health sector at a time when building national institutions in the public sector was the dominant creed. Problems surfaced in national health systems, however, as a consequence of overlooking economic efficiency and consumer satisfaction. Health interventions failed to reach their target populations, for instance, because the lack of drugs and unmotivated providers at clinics kept patients away, or because they provided services for which little consumer demand existed. Ignoring the importance of economic efficiency and consumer satisfaction also undermined the performance of health systems in the two dimensions that the planners sought to improve: equal access to low quality services led those who could to choose the private over the public sector; and poor incentives for providers negatively affected clinical effectiveness.

Evaluation of the Effectiveness of the Bank's Work in HNP

The previous section identified two elements or levers which influence the performance of health systems: institutional capacity and the demand-responsiveness of the structure of service delivery. That section also suggested four evaluative criteria against which to measure the performance of health systems, and which, in turn, determine the degree to which a health system directly influences changes in health outcomes. Building on this evaluative framework, this section further examines the pathways through which the Bank can influence health systems and health outcomes and discusses the methods to be used to evaluate the development effectiveness of the Bank's activities in the HNP sector.

The Bank is capable of influencing health systems and health outcomes through each of its three main activities—sector work and policy dialogue, investment, and evaluation. Sector work and policy dialogue can provide a diagnosis of a health system and its needs which can have a positive influence on the allocation of resources to the sector, project design, and project performance. The selection and appraisal of investments, as well as supervision, is the major activity through which the Bank directly affects health systems and health outcomes. The Bank's investment decisions with its clients encompass both direct investments in the structure or institutional capacity of a health system and those that work indirectly through changing socioeconomic status and household level demand for services. Last, the Bank's evaluation of its investments and lesson learning through monitoring project implementation and performance also contribute to improving its understanding of health systems and health outcomes.

The evaluation will span all three areas of World Bank work: policy dialogue and sector work, appraisal and supervision, and evaluation. The proposed study is divided into two distinct parts: (i) a broad and comparative assessment of the Bank's entire lending portfolio in HNP, and (ii) country sector impact studies that examine the World Bank's HNP relationship to several countries in detail. The rationale and methods for both parts follow.

Cross-country Analysis of Bank Lending

The evaluation will analyze the Bank's lending portfolio in HNP to provide a broad perspective on the Bank's activities and development effectiveness in the sector. Since most of the HNP portfolio consists of ongoing projects, the major component will be a comprehensive content analysis of Staff Appraisal Reports (SARs)[20]. This review of over 240 projects in 80 countries, covering FY80 to FY95, will examine the links between the quality of project design and likely development effectiveness. SARs will be evaluated on how they planned to strengthen institutional capacity and improve attentiveness to demand for the health system and their intended (implied) influence on system performance (clinical effectiveness, accessibility and equity, quality and consumer satisfaction, and economic efficiency). A focus on institutional capacity and attentiveness to consumer demand is unavoidable in this cross-country analysis, because on-going projects make up the bulk of the Bank's current HNP portfolio, and it is too early to judge their outcome. The review of SARs will also collect information on project content and design characteristics to provide a description of how Bank priorities and activities have evolved with time, stated project objectives, project components, and project costs.

Among the questions to be examined are the following:

- *What has been the scope of the Bank's project assistance? How have the objectives of HNP investments varied across country settings?*

20. Annex 5 presents the coding sheet to be used for coding the content of SARs for all completed and ongoing projects from FY80 to FY95.

- *What mechanisms do HNP projects employ to build flexibility into project implementation?*

- *What is the balance between efforts to establish or extend the health infrastructure and efforts to make the infrastructure effective in HNP project designs?*

- *Is complexity a necessary characteristic of HNP project design?*

- *What methods have projects employed to reach institutional development goals?*

- *How do HNP projects incorporate consumer views in the design of intervention programs?*

- *How well do HNP projects define and monitor the delivery of services to defined target populations?*

- *How is success defined?*

- *What mechanisms has the Bank employed to assure that it, and its Borrowers, are learning from the experience?*

For the quarter of the portfolio consisting of completed projects (n=60), the cross-country review will be supplemented by a review of how well the Bank has done in terms of development effectiveness, using, insofar as possible, the four criteria of (i) clinical effectiveness; (ii) accessibility and equity; (iii) consumer satisfaction; and (iv) economic efficiency. This review will be based on the Project Completion/Implementation Reports (PCRs and ICRs) supplemented by interviews with task managers.

To aid in the analysis, a database of socioeconomic indicators for the countries concerned will be constructed. This database will cover all 84 countries spanning the period FY80 to FY95 and contain country indicators representing both the health system as well as health status (life expectancy, total fertility rate (TFR), population per physician, etc.); social statistics (female and total secondary gross enrollment rates, female labor force as percent of total labor force, etc.); economic indicators (GDP per capita, annual domestic inflation, etc.); and governance indicators (political stability, bureaucratic delay, degree of corruption, etc.). This data will be extracted from the Bank's Economic and Social Database (BESD) for the years 1980-95, and will be supplemented by data on governance available in OED. This database will enable country level comparative analysis across income groups, health status, and by various macroeconomic indicators.

The cross-country analysis will also utilize information from the sixty completed projects to analyze implementation (supervision ratings, R_1) and outcomes (OED ratings, R_2) in relation to Bank inputs. These two ratings (R_1 and R_2), which will serve as dependent variables, will be predicted using as independent variables project characteristics such as design quality (D, indexed from the SAR data), project inputs (I, Bank and Borrower effort, staff weeks, and project costs), and societal determinants (S, including GDP and GDP growth, freedom from corruption, and other macroeconomic variables). The following equation will be estimated:

$$R_n = f(D, I, S)$$

The results from this reduced form equation, estimated separately for supervision ratings and project outcomes, are intended to offer insights into several issues: whether effective project implementation (and outcome) depends mainly on vectors measuring societal factors (S) beyond the reach of the project itself; whether it depends, to the contrary, on particular features of project design (D), which tend to be the focus of attention within the sector; and/or whether it depends on inputs such as Bank and Borrower effort (I) which might complement or negate the effects of good design.

Country Sector Impact Studies

As argued above, development is effective in health care only if it makes people healthier; but because the data on mortality and morbidity rates in the developing world are inadequate and because the causes of good health are not fully understood, attributing changes in health status to specific World Bank interventions would not be credible. Rather, in evaluating development effectiveness, plausible links must be established across the sequence of development interventions. A cross-country analysis is not suited to such a task. Instead, in depth examinations of individual countries are needed. These country studies will examine the effects of projects and non-lending interventions on health system institutional capacity, the demand-responsiveness of the structure of service delivery, and changed patterns of demand. They will then look for plausible connections between changes in health care delivery systems as a result of Bank interventions and changes in the four measures of health system performance: (i) clinical/epidemiological effectiveness; (ii) accessibility and equity; (iii) perceived quality and consumer satisfaction; and iv) economic efficiency. The data for measuring development effectiveness along these four dimensions will not always be complete or comparable, nor will it be easy to isolate the effect of the World Bank's work from the activities of governments and other donors.

Even in countries with advanced health care systems, *clinical/epidemiological effectiveness* is notoriously difficult to define and to measure. The country studies will not attempt direct assessment (which would at a minimum require detailed outcome data) but will focus on the clinical appropriateness (according to current standards of medical care and epidemiological effectiveness) of the menu of goods and services provided by the health care system. An assessment will be made of how up-to-date and locally appropriate available goods and services are for a number of health conditions, especially those of greatest epidemiological significance in the country studied. The degree to which health providers (private as well as public) are properly trained and equipped to provide appropriate care will also be assessed. To the extent possible, this assessment will be both current and retrospective, to see whether Bank advice and Bank projects have improved the menu of goods and services and the ability to provide them. Some information will come from available reviews of health care and status in the particular country, such as previous Bank sector reviews, and additional information will be obtained in interviews or from focus groups of providers, medical educators, and public and private health officials.

Standards of care vary considerably within most developing countries, and questions of *access and equity* therefore require careful attention. A variety of measures of access should exist in most countries, such as numbers of facilities and providers per capita, and utilization rates of specific health services in the public, private, and traditional sectors. Breaking these data down according to income class, geographic location, gender, and ethnic group will provide measures of equity. To supplement these data and better describe the current situation, both on the access and equity sides, a questionnaire on service availability and utilization (Annex 2) will be administered to knowledgeable government officials and health services staff, small groups of private providers, representatives of NGOs and to Bank staff and other donor staff in each country studied.

A second important approach to questions of equity and access will be the analysis of survey data on household health-related experiences and behavior. Such data are available in a few countries from surveys, such as the Living Standard Measurement Survey (LSMS) and the Demographic and Health Status Survey (DHS). The main questions to be tackled in using these data will be how access to and utilization of services vary cross-sectionally and how and why the pattern has changed over time and, wherever possible, an examination of possible links to particular project activities. These data will be supplemented by review of reports of service utilization from ongoing service statistics and monitoring and evaluation (M&E) systems where these data are available and sufficiently reliable to allow analysis.

Household surveys may also provide measures of perceived *quality and consumer satisfaction*. Other available polls, surveys, and beneficiary assessments will also be consulted. Where possible, new surveys or focus groups involving actual and intended beneficiaries of Bank projects will be conducted. These inquiries will cover actual beneficiary utilization of services (from all sources—traditional, private, and public); beneficiaries' appraisals of providers, facilities, and the treatment they received; their judgments about how services have changed; and their recommendations for improving services.

Evaluations of the *economic efficiency* of the health care system will not be precise because the systematic use of cost-effectiveness and other forms of economic analysis in the sector is relatively new. Nevertheless, reviews of sector work, public expenditure reviews, and other documents and interviews with key officials should help provide answers to questions such as the following:

- *Did World Bank policy dialogue and lending direct government attention to areas with substantial public goods or externalities?*

- *Were the funded projects high on a list of the most cost-effective interventions? Was any cost-effectiveness analysis completed during project preparation?*

- *Did World Bank activities promote the most efficient provider-reimbursement systems available in the countries? Did they encourage regulation of the insurance market to redress market failures?*

- *Did World Bank sectoral reform efforts promote taxation for health care services and medical user fees in the most efficiency-enhancing and equitable manner, given the countries' political and institutional situation?*

The standards against which health projects can be judged have changed over time (in fact, are currently very much a matter of debate), in response to changes in medical and public health technology (or state of the art), as well as in response to much recent analysis in such areas as the cost-effectiveness of different interventions, and emerging views on the role of public finance in the health sector. Assessing past Bank efforts against current standards, building on recent work completed by HDD (Preker, Brenzel, and Atta 1996) should help to find ways in which the Bank can improve its work.

The assessment of health care system performance using the four criteria given will be supplemented by an assessment of the Bank's effects on the health system's institutional capacity and demand sensitivity. Beyond an inventory of facilities, staff and programs, this will require a look behind the scenes at such things as the information and planning system, the incentive system for providers, political support for health care, and other "rules of the game" that determine what resources the health care system can command and how they are deployed. Existing documents and interviews with key officials and Bank staff will be the main sources of information, to be supplemented with a questionnaire for the key informants themselves on institutional development and sustainability issues.

In sum, the country studies will rely on a review of previous Bank reports and other documents on the health system and assembly of health data from household surveys and other sources and some re-analysis of such data where appropriate. In addition, the studies will employ beneficiary surveys or focus groups where feasible, interviews and focus groups involving health providers, health officials, Bank staff, and other donor staff, and questionnaires for some of these key informants to assess performance of the health system. Wherever reliable trend data on health outcomes can be identified, such as data on particular disease conditions, or particular forms of mortality targeted by a Bank project, these too will be utilized with a view to delineating the counterfactual: How would the health system have performed in the absence of Bank intervention?

The working hypothesis underlying these studies is that incentive structures and the other elements of the economic organization of health delivery systems, particularly their institutional capacity and their attentiveness to demand, are the critical pathways through which World Bank interventions can best improve the performance of health systems. In other words, where Bank project designs and supervision missions utilize carefully developed analyses of institutional capacity, health care systems will exhibit the most improvement when measured by the four nominated evaluative criteria. To test this hypothesis, each country study will also characterize the institutional capacity and the institutional development of the countries' health care systems.[21]

Country Selection

Because the studies will be complex descriptive accounts in which statistical comparisons will not be complete or decisive, a random sample of countries would probably obscure more information than it revealed. Rather, the countries will be purposively in accord with specific criteria.

First, all or most of the countries should have had substantial interaction with the World Bank in the health care sector. The direct goal of the study is to evaluate the development

---

21. A questionnaire on institutional development has been prepared based on the work of Bernhardt (1992). Questions cover (i) planning (epidemiological knowledge, estimates of demand, targets or goals, monitoring, and budgeting); (ii) client orientation (utilization, consumer feedback, and consumer satisfaction); (iii) staffing issues (incentives, skill development, and evaluation of performance); (iv) management (data and logistics); (v) field supervision; (vi) management's ability to determine and control costs; and (vii) problem solving ability (see Annex 3).

effectiveness of the Bank's work in the field, not simply to identify best practice strategies. This requires countries where the World Bank has played a substantial role. These countries might be those with a substantial volume of borrowing (India, Indonesia, Brazil), with a record of borrowing and/or policy dialogue that spans most of the decade and a half of World Bank involvement in HNP (India, Indonesia), or in which the ratio of Bank lending to country expenditures in the sector is relatively high (Zimbabwe, Uganda, Côte d'Ivoire).

Second, the countries selected should span one or more stages of the "epidemiological transition." A number of developing countries are moving from an epidemiological profile with high rates of communicable disease transmission, infant mortality, and fertility to a profile in which the leading causes of death will soon be non-communicable, such as heart disease, cancer, and accidents (Chile, Malaysia). Other countries are still far from that transition (Bolivia, Nepal), and several are sharply dual, with an industrialized country profile in the cities alongside high prevalence of communicable diseases and infant mortality among rural populations and urban slum dwellers (Mexico, India). Countries at different stages of this transition encounter distinct sets of problems and demand different kinds of interventions.

Third, the countries should exhibit variation in the characteristics of their health care delivery systems, including variation in the mode of health care delivery. Some countries have systems that emphasize expensive clinical care in large urban hospitals (Zambia), and others focus on public health concerns and primary care (the Gambia). Some countries have centralized systems (Indonesia), and others have devolved authority to localities or provinces (Chile). The private sector is widely utilized in some countries, either in the form of modern for-profit physicians (Thailand) or traditional healers and households (Sudan), and in others the public sector dominates health care (Nicaragua). Comparing countries across these axes of variation may permit the institutional structures most conducive to successful interventions to be identified.

Fourth, at least two, and perhaps most, of the countries chosen should have had experience with both disease-specific projects and World Bank-assisted sectoral reform. The balance of Bank lending and sectoral strategy in recent years has shifted from disease-specific interventions and the construction of new facilities to the reform of policymaking institutions in health care. Examining countries with both kinds of "projects" will permit an evaluation of the relative benefits of the two strategies and the factors associated with their performance.

Finally, the set of countries should be balanced across regions and should not focus exclusively on either large or small countries. Focusing on one or two regions might lead to mistaking the historical experiences of one or two sets of countries or of one or two departments of the World Bank, for that matter, for general lessons. Including both large and small countries is also important because the size of a country might be inversely related to the extent of the World Bank's influence on their HNP policies, one of the study's chief areas of concern.

Annex 4 lists demographic, health system, and project characteristics for all countries that have borrowed in the HNP sector. From that universe, those countries that have had substantial interaction with the World Bank measured by the relative volume of their borrowing, the absolute volume of their borrowing, or the length of their policy dialogue, and those with both disease-specific and systemic reform projects—in other words, countries that satisfy criteria one and four above—have been selected and are listed separately in Table 5.1. Table 5.1 also characterizes the broad epidemiological status of the countries (based on the data in Annex 4), used in criterion two, and the dominant subsector in the area of health care (based on relative expenditures), an element of criterion three. Although the structure and function of the countries' health delivery systems are also interesting axes of variation, the degree of decentralization in a country's medical system and the emphasis it places on primary care is too complex to capture in the table. These are traits intimately connected to the particular history of each country, and each country sector impact study will find informative variation in those areas.

Three country clusters have been identified based on these criteria: Cluster 1: Jamaica, Indonesia, India, Zimbabwe, and Malawi; Cluster 2: Colombia, Indonesia, India, Zimbabwe, and Mali; and Cluster 3: Brazil, Zimbabwe, China, India, and Uganda. Five countries will finally be selected from these clusters.

Table 5.1: Traits of Countries with Substantial Interaction with the World Bank in both Disease-specific Projects and Health Policy Reform

	Number of projects (closed, active)	Stage in epidemiological transition	Dominant sector
LAC			
Argentina	0,2	Late	Public
Brazil	4,5	Middle	Public
Colombia	2,2	Middle	Even
Jamaica	2,2	Late	Public
Venezuela	0,3	Late	Public
MENA			
Morocco	1,1	Middle	Private
Tunisia	2,2	Middle	Public
Yemen	2,4	Early	Private
EAST ASIA			
China	1,5	Middle	Public
Indonesia	8,4	Middle	Private
Philippines	2,3	Middle	Even
SOUTH ASIA			
Bangladesh	3,2	Early	Private
India	6,13	Early	Private
Pakistan	1,3	Early	Even
Sri Lanka	0,2	Late	Even
ECA			
Turkey	0,2	Middle	Private
AFRICA			
Burkina Faso	0,3	Early	Private
Malawi	2,1	Early	Even
Mali	1,1	Early	Private
Nigeria	1,4	Early	Private
Uganda	0,4	Early	Private
Zimbabwe	1,2	Middle	Even

Source: Author's calculations.

Summary

This chapter has presented the elements of a proposed assessment of the development effectiveness of the Bank's HNP activities. The design of this evaluation draws on the findings presented in chapters 1-4 which reviewed the literature on health and fertility transitions, previous efforts to evaluate health policies and programs, as well as existing assessments of the Bank's experience in HNP. An evaluative framework for studying health systems has been outlined which suggests that the study focus on an assessment of the Bank's experiences in influencing the demand responsiveness of service delivery structures and institutional capacity in borrower settings and the development effectiveness of these efforts measured against four criteria: clinical effectiveness, accessibility and equity, economic efficiency, and the degree of consumer satisfaction with health care services.

The evaluation will span all three areas of World Bank work: policy dialogue and sector work, investment, and evaluation. The proposed study method has two parts: country studies and a cross-country comparative analysis.

The combination of the country impact studies and the cross-country analysis will yield insights as to the factors important for health system performance, potentially suggesting various ways of increasing the impact of projects and improving development effectiveness. This study will also initiate a new discussion of the significance for development effectiveness. the study will also initiate a new discussion of the significance for development of HNP projects. Health has often been considered a paramount good, and attempts to improve it seem self-evidently worthwhile. But the increasing financial burden of health care systems and the growing possibilities for improving health outcomes at relatively low cost suggest that more critical evaluations could be of considerable benefit.

References

AID (Agency for International Development). 1978. "Demonstration and Evaluation: Public Health, Ethiopia." Washington, D.C.

———. 1979. *Determinants of Fertility Change*. Washington, D.C.

———. 1981. "Housing and Health: An Analysis for Use in the Planning, Design, and Evaluation of Low-Income Housing Programs." Office of Housing and Urban Development. Washington, D.C.

———. 1990. "Factors Influencing the Sustainability of U.S. Foreign Assistance Programs in Health 1942–1989: A Six Country Synthesis." AID Evaluation Working Paper Report No. 149. Washington, D.C.

Akin, John S., Charles C. Griffin, David K. Guilkey, and Barry M. Popkin. 1986. "The Demand for Primary Health Care Services in the Bicol Region of the Philippines." *Economic Development and Cultural Change* 34(4): 755–82.

Alderman, Harold. 1994. "Research as an Input into Nutrition Policy Formation." World Bank Human Resources Development and Operations Policy Working Paper 32. Washington, D.C.

Alderman, Harold and Victor Lavy. 1996. "Household Responses to Public Health Services: Cost and Quality Tradeoffs." *World Bank Research Observer* 11(1):3-22.

American Public Health Association and U.S. Agency for International Development. 1979. "Thailand National Family Planning Program Evaluation: A Report." Office of Population. Washington, D.C.

Amin, Ruhul, Shifiq A. Chowdhury, G. M. Kamal, and J. Chowdhury. 1990. "Community Health Services and Health Care Utilization in Rural Bangladesh." *Social Science and Medicine* 29(12):1343–49.

Anker, M. 1993. "Rapid Evaluation Methods (REM) in Health Services Performance: Methodological Observation." *Bulletin of the World Health Organization* 71(1):15–21.

Arias, Oscar. 1995. "Results of the Country Economic Analysis for the Annual Review of Evaluation Results, 1994." OED Working Paper. World Bank, Washington, D.C.

Aziz, K., and others. 1990. *Water Supply, Sanitation and Hygiene Education: Report of a Health Impact Study in Mirzapur, Bangladesh*. UNDP-World Bank Water and Sanitation Program, Water and Sanitation Report Series 1. Washington, D.C.: World Bank.

Baldwin, George. 1992. "Targets and Indicators in Population Projects." Policy Research Working Paper WPS 1048. World Bank, Population, Health and Nutrition Department, Washington, D.C.

Barutwanayo, Marianne, and others. 1993. "Malaria Control in Africa: Guidelines for the Evaluation National Programs." Atlanta, Ga.: U.S. Public Health Service, Centers for Disease Control and Prevention.

Beegle, Kathleen. 1994. "The Quality and Availability of Family Planning Services and Contraceptive Use in Tanzania." Michigan State University. Photocopy.

Berelson, Bernard. 1978. *Programs and Prospects for Fertility Reduction: What? Where?* Population Council Working Paper 31. New York.

Berelson, Bernard, and Ronald Freedman. 1976. "A Review of the Implementation of the Recommendations of the External Advisory Committee on Population. External Review." World Bank, Washington, D.C. Photocopy.

Berg, Alan. 1980. *Nutrition, Basic Needs and Growth*. Washington, D.C.: World Bank.

———. 1987. *Malnutrition. What Can Be Done? Lessons from World Bank Experience*. Baltimore: Johns Hopkins University Press for the World Bank.

———. 1994. *Enriching Lives. Overcoming Vitamin and Mineral Malnutrition in Developing Countries*. Washington, D.C.: World Bank.

Berman, Peter, and Laura Rose. 1994. *The Role of Private Providers in Maternal and Child Health and Family Planning Services in Developing Countries*. Cambridge, Mass.: Harvard School of Public Health.

Bernhart, Michael H. 1992. "Sustainability: An Interactive Assessment Program." PC/Windows Version 1.3. University Research Corporation.

Bertrand, Jane T., Robert J. Magnani, and James C. Knowles. 1994. *Handbook of Indicators for Family Planning Program Evaluation*. The Evaluation Project. Chapel Hill, N.C.: University of North Carolina.

Bhatia, Shushum, F. Saadah, and W. H. Moseley. "Analytical Review of the Development of Family Planning Program Strategies, Operations, and Research as Model for Primary Health Care Programs." Paper prepared for the International Commission on Health Research for Development. Johns Hopkins School of Hygiene and Public Health, Department of Population Dynamics, Baltimore, Md.

Birdsall, Nancy. 1989. "Thoughts on Good health and Good Government." *Daedalus* 118(Winter):89–124.

———. 1992. "Pragmatism, Robin Hood and Other Themes: Good Government and Social Well Being in Developing Countries." In Chen and others, *Social Dimensions of Transition*.

Birdsall, Nancy, ed. 1983. *The Effects of Family Planning Programs on Fertility in the Developing World*. Working Paper 677, Series Number 2. World Bank, Population and Development, Washington, D.C.

Birdsall, Nancy, and Robert Hecht. 1995. *Swimming Against the Tide: Strategies for Improving Equity in Health*. World Bank, Human Resources Development and Operations Policy, Working Paper Number 55. Washington, D.C.

Birdsall, Nancy, and Estelle James. 1990. *Efficiency and Equity in Social Spending: How and Why Governments Misbehave*. Working Paper 274. World Bank, Population and Human Resources Operations Department,. Washington, D.C.

———. 1994. "Health, Government, and the Poor: The Case for the Private Sector." In James N. Gribble and Samuel H. Preston, eds., *The Epidemiological Transition: Policy and Planning Implications for Developing Countries*. Washington, D.C.: National Academy Press.

Bloom, Abby L. 1984. "Prospects for Primary Health Care in Africa: Another Look at the Sine Saloum Rural Health Project in Senegal." Evaluation Special Study No. 20. Washington, D.C.: U.S. Agency for International Development.

Bobadilla, José-Luis, and Peter Cowley. 1995. "Designing and Implementing Packages of Essential Health Services." *Journal of International Development* 7(3):543–54.

Bobadilla, José-Luis, J. Frenk, T. Frejka, R. Lozano, and C. Stern. 1993. "The Epidemiological Transition and Health Sector Priorities." In Dean T. Jamison and W. H. Mosley, eds., *Disease Control Priorities in Developing Countries*.New York: Oxford University Press for the World Bank.

Bobadilla, José-Luis, and Cristin de A. Possas. 1994. "Health Policy Issues in Three Latin American Countries: Implications of the Epidemiological Transition." In James N. Gribble and Samuel H. Preston, eds., *The Epidemiological Transition: Policy and Planning Implications for Developing Countries*. Washington, D.C.: National Academy Press..

Bongaarts, John. 1978. "A Framework for Analyzing the Proximate Determinants of Fertility." *Population and Development Review* 4:105–32.

———. 1985. *The Role of Family Planning Programs in Contemporary Fertility Transitions*. Population Council Research Division Working Paper 71. New York.

———. 1994. "The Impact of Population Policies: Comment." *Population and Development* 20(3):616–20.

Boque, Donald J. 1969. *Principles of Demography*. New York: John Wiley and Sons.

Boulier, Bryan L. 1983. "Family Planning Programs and Contraceptive Availability: Their Effects on Contraceptive Use and Fertility." In Nancy Birdsall, ed., *The Effects of Family*

Planning Programs on Fertility in the Developing World. Working Paper 677, Series Number 2. World Bank, Population and Development, Washington, D.C.

Boyd, Derick. 1987. "Appraisal of District Level Resource Utilization of Primary Health Care: A Case Study of Christian Pen, Jamaica." University of West Indies, Mona, Kingston, Jamaica.

Brinkerhoff, Derick W. 1994. "Institutional Development in World Bank Projects: Analytical Appoaches and Intervention Designs." *Public Administration and Development* 14:135–51.

Buckner, Bates, Amy Tsui, Albert Hermalin, and Catherine McKaig, eds. 1995. *A Guide to Methods of Family Planning Program Evaluation, 1965-1990.* The Evaluation Project. Chapel Hill, N.C.: University of North Carolina.

Bulatao, Rodolfo. 1993. *Effective Family Planning Programs.* Washington, D.C.: World Bank.

———. 1995. *Key Indicators for Family Planning Projects.* World Bank Technical Paper 297. Washington, D.C.

———. 1996. "Dissecting Family Planning Sustainability." Photocopy.

Bulatao, Rudolpho, and Laura B. Shrestha. 1995. "Key Indicators for Reproductive Health Projects." Mimeo. World Bank, Population, Health, and Nutrition Department, Washington, D.C.

Burkhardt, Robert, and others. 1980. "Family Planning in Rural Egypt: A View From the Health System." TAP Report, Monograph/M.I.T.–Cairo University Health Care Delivery Systems Project #6. Cambridge, Mass.: Massachusetts Institute of Technology.

Caldwell, John C. 1986. "Routes to Low Mortality in Poor Countries." *Population and Development Review* 12(2):171–220.

Caldwell, John, Sally Findley, and others. 1990. "What We Know about Health Transition: The Cultural, Social and Behavioral Determinants of Health. Volumes I and II." The Proceedings of an International Workshop, Canberra. Australian National University Press.

Carrin, Guy. 1984. *Economic Evaluation of Health Care in Developing Countries: Theory and Applications.* London: C. Helm; New York: St. Martin's.

Chen, Lincoln C., and Richard A. Cash. 1988. "A Decade after Alma Ata: Can Primary Health Care Lead to Health for All?" *The New England Journal of Medicine* 319(14):946–47.

Chaudhri, Rajiv, and C. Peter Timmer. 1986. "The Impact of Changing Affluence on Diet and Demand Patterns for Agricultural Commodities." Working Paper 785. World Bank, Washington, D.C.

Chowdury, Shafiq A. 1986. "Determinants of Health Care Utilization in Rural Bangladesh." *PRICOR. Primary Health Care Operations Research* 35:1–2.

Cochrane, Susan H. 1979. "Fertility and Education: What Do We Really Know?" Washington, D.C.: World Bank.

Cochrane, Susan H., Donald J. O'Hara, and Joann Leslie. "The Effects of Education on Health." Working Paper 405. World Bank, Washington, D.C.

Cohen, Paul, and John Purcal, eds. 1989. *The Political Economy of Primary Health Care in Southeast Asia*. Canberra: Australian Development Studies Network.

Coleman, Gilroy. 1993. "Evaluating the Health Impact of Water and Sanitation Projects: It Ain't Necessarily Necessary." *Project Appraisal* 8:251–55.

Commission on Health Research for Development. 1990. *Health Research: Essential Link to Equity in Development*. Oxford, U.K.: Oxford University Press.

Cooper Weill, D. E., A. P. Alicbusan, J. F. Wilson, and others. 1990. "The Impact of Development Policies on Health: A Review of the Literature." Geneva: WHO.

Coppedge, Michael, and Wolfgang H. Reinke. 1990. Measuring Polyarchy." *Studies in Comparative International Development* 25(1):51-72.

Courtois, Xavier, and Jerome Dumoulin. 1995. "Sale of Drugs and Health Care Utilization in a Health Care District in Zaire." *Health Policy and Planning* 10:181–85.

Cropper, Maureen L., and Uma Subramanian. 1995. "Public Choices between Lifesaving Programs." Policy Research Working Paper 1497. World Bank, Environment, Infrastructure and Agriculture Division, Policy Research Department and Asia Technical Department Environment and Natural Resources Division, Washington, D.C.

Cubbon, John E. 1987. "Methods of Evaluating Community Health Services at Local Level: Possible Applications of Routinely Collected Data." *Community Medicine* 9(4)323–30.

Cuca, Roberto, and Catherine Pierce. 1977. *Experiments in Family Planning: Lessons from the Developing World*. Baltimore: Johns Hopkins University Press for the World Bank.

Deboeck, G. 1980. *Systems for Monitoring and Evaluating Nutritional Interventions*. Washington, D.C.: World Bank.

De Geyndt, Willy. 1995. "Managing the Quality of Health Care in Developing Countries." World Bank Technical Paper 258. Washington, D.C.

Diwan, Vinod Kumar. 1992. *Epidemiology in Context: Effectiveness of Health Care Interventions*. Stockholm: Karolinska Institutet.

Dunlop, D. 1980. "Health Project Evaluation: Economic and Social Issues." Paper prepared for Inter-American Development Bank Seminar on Health Project Impacts. Washington, D.C. Photocopy.

Dunlop, David W., and USAID. 1982. "Toward a Health Project Evaluation Framework." AID Evaluation Special Study No. 8. Washington, D.C.

The Economist. 1995. "Good Intentions, Road to Hell?" October 7 , p. 91.

Elmendorf, A. Edward, and Chastain Fitzgerald. 1995. "Lessons Learned from Experience in World Bank Population, Health and Nutrition Projects in Africa: A Synthesis of Implementation Completion Reports." World Bank, Africa Technical Department, Human Resources and Poverty Division. Washington, D.C. Processed.

Engelkes, Elly. 1990. "Process Evaluation in Colombian Primary Health Care Programme." Health Policy and Planning 5:327–35.

Engelkes, P. E. M. 1989. Health For All?: Evaluation and Monitoring in a Comprehensive Primary Health Care Project in Columbia. Amsterdam, Netherlands: Royal Tropical Institute.

———. 1992. "Evaluation of Community Health Services Utilization." Tropical and Geographical Medicine 44: 52–57.

The Evaluation Project. 1992. "Expert Meeting on Future Needs for Evaluating Family Planning Programs, September 11, 1992." Chapel Hill, N.C.

———. 1993a. "Indicators of Quality of Care in International Family Planning Programs." Chapel Hill, N.C.

———. 1993b. "Seminar on Cost Analysis Service Delivery Working Group: Minutes of Meeting, September 13–14, 1993." Chapel Hill, N.C.

Faruqee, Rashid. 1982. Analyzing the Impact of Health Services: Project Experience from India, Ghana, and Thailand. World Bank Working Paper 546. Washington, D.C.

Feachem, R. G. A., and Dean T. Jamison. 1991. Disease and Mortality in Sub-Saharan Africa. New York: Oxford University Press for the World Bank.

Feachem, R. G. A., T. Kjellstrom, C. J. L. Murray,, M. Over, and M. Philips, eds. 1992. The Health of Adults in the Developing World. New York: Oxford University Press for the World Bank.

Feifer, Chris Naschak. 1990. "Maternal Health in Jamaica: Health Needs, Services, and Utilization." Policy Research Working Paper 539. World Bank, Washington, D.C.

Fisher, Andrew, Barbara Mensch, Robert Miller, Ian Askew, Anrudh Jain, Cecilia Ndeti, Lewis Ndhlovu, and Placide Tapsoba. 1992. "Guidelines and Instruments for a Family Planning Situation Analysis Study." Africa Operations Research and Technical Assistance Project

73

and the Robert H. Ebert Program on Critical Issues in Reproductive Health and Population. New York: The Population Council.

Foreit, Karen G., and J. R. Foreit, G. Lagos, and A. Guzman. 1993. "Effectiveness and Cost-Effectiveness of Postpartum IUD Insertion in Lima, Peru." *Inernational Family Planning Perspectives* (19(1):19-24.

Forman, Martin J., ed. 1986. *Nutritional Aspects of Project Food Aid.* Rome: United Nations.

Foster, S. 1979. "Monitoring Health for All." Paper prepared for World Health Organization. Washington, D.C. Photocopy.

Freedman, Deborah S., and R. Freedman. 1986. "Adding Demand-Side Variables to Study the Interaction Between Demand and Supply in Bangladesh." Population, Health and Nutrition Technical Note 86-28. Washington, D.C.: World Bank.

Freedman, Ronald, and B. Berelson. 1978. "Conditions of Fertility Decline in Developing Countries, 1965–1975." *Studies in Family Planning* 9:89–148.

Freedman, Ronald, and J. Y. Takeshita. 1969. *Family Planning in Taiwan: An Experiment in Social Change.* Princeton, N.J.: Princeton University Press.

Ganatra, B., and S. Hirve. 1994. "Male Bias in Health Care Utilization for Under-Fives in a Rural Community in Western India." *World Health Organization Bulletin* 72(1):101–4.

Garcia-Nunez, Jose. 1992. *Improving Family Planning Evaluation: A Step-by-Step Guide for Managers and Evaluators.* West Hartford, Conn.: Kumarian.

Gastil, Raymond. 1987. *Freedom in the World: Political Rights and Civil Liberties.* New York: Greenwood Press.

Gertler, Paul J., and John W. Molyneaux. 1994. "How Economic Development and Family Planning Programs Combined to Reduce Indonesian Fertility." *Demography* 31(1):33–63.

Gertler, P., L. Locay, W. Sanderson, A. Dor, and J. van der Gaag. 1988. "Health Care Financing and the Demand for Medical Care." Living Standards Measurement Study Working Paper 37. World Bank, Washington, D.C.

Ghana Health Assessment Project Team. 1981. "A Quantitative Method of Assessing the Health Impact of Different Diseases in Less Developed Countries." *International Journal of Epidemiology* 10(1):73–80.

Gish, Oscar. 1990. "Some Links Between Successful Implementation of Primary Health Care Interventions and the Overall Utilization of Health Services." *Social Science and Medicine* 30(4):401–5.

———.1995. "Health Service Utilization as a Measure of Needs Equity and Resource Allocation." WHO Expert Review of Health Research and Development Priorities.

Gish, Oscar, Ridwan Malik, and Paramita Suharto. 1988. "Who Gets What? Utilization of Health Services in Indonesia." *International Journal of Health Planning and Management* 3:185–96.

Gomez, Luis Carlos. 1988. "Household Survey of Health Services Utilization in Santo Domingo, Dominican Republic." In *Health Care Financing in Latin America and the Caribbean: Research Report 8.* Stony Brook, N.Y.: State University of New York at Stony Brook.

Gribble, James N., and Samuel H. Preston, eds. 1993. *The Epidemiological Transition: Policy and Planning Implications for Developing Countries.* Committee on Population, National Research Council. Washington, D.C.:National Academy Press.

Griffin, Charles C. 1992. *Health Care in Asia. A Comparative Study of Cost and Financing.* Washington, D.C.: World Bank.

Grindle, Merilee S., and John W. Thomas. 1991. *Public Choices and Policy Change: The Political Economy of Reform in Developing Countries.* Baltimore, Md.: The Johns Hopkins University Press.

Grosh, Margaret E., and Paul Glewwe. 1995. *A Guide to Living Standards Measurement Study Surveys and Their Data Sets.* Living Standards Measurement Study Working Paper 120. World Banmk, Washington, D.C.

Grossman, Jean Baldwin. 1994. "Evaluating Social Policies: Principles and U.S. Experience." *The World Bank Research Observer* 9(2):159–80.

Guerra, Raineri, and International Course for Primary Health Care Managers at District Level in Developing Countries. 1991. *Global Evaluation, Joint WHO-UNICEF Nutrition Support Programme.* Rome: International Course for Primary Health Care Managers at District Level in Developing Countries.

Guerrero, Rodrigo. 1995. "The Task Force for Child Survival and Development: An Evaluation." Mimeo. Washington, D.C. Photocopy.

Gustafson, Daniel J. 1994. "Developing Sustainable Institutions; Lessons from Cross-case Analysis of 24 Agricultural Extension Programs." *Public Administration and Development* 14:121–34.

Gwatkin, David, and J. Wray. 1980. "Can Health and Nutrition Interventions Make a Difference." Washington, D.C.: Overseas Development Council.

Haddad, Lawrence, and S. M. Ravi Kanbur. 1991. "The Value of Intra-Household Survey Data for Age-Based Nutritional Targeting." Policy, Research and External Affairs Working Paper 684. World Bank, Washington, D.C.

Haddad, Slim, and Pierre Fournier. 1995. "Quality, Cost and Utilization of Health Services in Developing Countries: A Longitudinal Study in Zaire." *Social Science and Medicine* 40(6):743–53.

Halstead, Scott B., Julia Walsh, and Kenneth Warren. 1985. *Good Health at Low Cost.* Conference Report. Rockefeller Foundation. New York.

Harvard Institute for International Development. 1981. "Nutrition Intervention in Developing Countries, Study VII, Integrated Nutrition and Primary Health Care Programs." Cambridge, Mass.

Heaver, Richard. 1984. "Adapting the Training and Visit System for Family Planning, Health, and Nutrition Programs." Staff Working Paper 662. World Bank, Washington, D.C.

———. 1988. "Reaching People at the Periphery: Can the World Bank's Population, Health, and Nutrition Operations do Better?" Working Paper Series 81. World Bank, Population and Human Resources Department, Washington, D.C.

———. 1991a. "Participative Rural Appraisal: Potential Applications to Family Planning, Health and Nutrition Programs." World Bank, Asia Technical Department. Washington, D.C.

———. 1991b. "Using Field Visits to Improve the Quality of Family Planning, Health, and Nutrition Programs: A Supervisor's Manual." Washington, D.C.: World Bank.

Heller, P. S. 1982. "A Model of the Demand for Medical and Health Services in Peninsular Malaysia." *Social Science and Medicine* 16:267.

Henderson, Gail, and others. 1994. "Equity and Utilization of Health Services: Report of an Eight-Province Survey in China." *Social Science and Medicine* 39(5):687–99.

Herz, Barbara, K. Subbarao, Masooma Habib, and Laura Raney. 1991. *Letting Girls Learn: Promising Approaches in Primary and Secondary Education.* World Bank Discussion Paper 133. Washington, D.C.

Holland, Walter W., ed. 1983. *Evaluation of Health Care.* Sponsored by the Commission of the European Communities. New York: Oxford University Press.

Horton, Susan. 1991. "Unit-costs, Cost-Effectiveness, and Financing of Nutrition Interventions." Working Paper Series 952. World Bank, Population and Human Resources Department, Washington, D.C.

Institute for Resource Development/Macro Systems, Peru. 1989. *Experimental Study: An Evaluation of Fertility and Child Health Information.* Princeton, N.J.: Princeton University Press.

IADB (Inter-American Development Bank). 1988. "Summary of the Ex-Post Evaluations of Public Health Programs." Office of the Controller, Operations Evaluations Office, Washington, D.C.

International Institute for the Study of Human Reproduction, Center for Population and Family Health, and U.S. Agency for International Development. 1990. "Program Planning

Management Review and Evaluation Accounting Contraceptives Oral Rehydration Therapy Immunization Survey Methodology Sampling Microcomputers." New York, N.Y.: Center for Population and Family Health.

Jamison, Dean. 1985. "China's Health Care System: Policies, Organization, Inputs and Finance." In Halsted, Walsh, and Warren, eds., *Good Health at Low Cost*.

Jamison, Dean T., W. Mosley, A. R. Measham, and J. Bobadilla, eds. 1993. *Disease Control Priorities in Developing Countries*. New York: Oxford University Press for the World Bank.

Janowitz, Barbara, and J. Bratt. 1994. *Methods for Costing Family Planning Services*. United Nations Fund for Population Activities and Family Health International. New York.

Kaufman, Daniel and Yan Wang. 1992. "How Macroeconomic Policies Affect Project Performance in the Social Sectors." Policy Research Working Papaers 939. Washington, D.C.: World Bank.

Keling, R, and others. 1979. *Evaluating the Impact of Nutrition and Health Programs*. Washington, D.C.

Kennedy, Eileen T. 1991. "Successful Nutrition Programs in Africa: What Makes Them Work?" Working Paper 706. World Bank, Population and Human Resources Department. Washington, D.C.

Khalifa, Atef M., and others. 1981. "An Evaluation of the Impact of the Population and Development Program (PDP)." Agency for International Development, Office of Population and Westinghouse Health Systems and Contraceptive Prevalence Survey Project. Cairo: Population and Family Planning Board.

Kielman, Arnfried A., and Associates. 1983. *Child and Maternal Health Services in Rural India: The Narangwal Experiment. Volume I. Integrated Nutrition and Health Care*. Baltimore, Md.: The Johns Hopkins University Press for the World Bank.

King, Timothy, and others. 1974. *Population Policies and Economic Development*. Baltimore, Md.: The Johns Hopkins University Press for the World Bank.

Klein, Robert E., and others. 1979. *Evaluating the Impact of Nutrition and Health Programs*. New York: Plenum.

Kloos, Helmut. 1990. "Utilization of Selected Hospitals, Health Centres and Health Stations in Central, Southern and Western Ethiopia." *Social Science and Medicine* 31(2):101–15.

Koenig, M., V. Fauveau, A. Chowdhury, J. Chakraboty, and M. Khan. 1988. "Maternal Mortality in Matlab, Bangladesh: 1975-1985." *Studies in Family Planning* 19(2):69–80.

Kohn, Robert, and Kerr L. White. 1976. *Health Care: An International Study: Report of the World Health Organization/International Collaborative Study of Medical Care Utilization*. New York: Oxford University Press.

Kuhner, A. 1971. "The Impact of Public Health Programs on Economic Development: report of a Study of Malaria in Thailand." *International Journal of Health Services* 1(3).

Kumar, A., K. Shiva, and Vanita Nayak Mukherjee. 1993. "Health as Development: Implications for Research, Policy, and Action." *Economic and Political Weekly* 28:769–74.

Kunitz, Stephen J., and Stanley L. Engerman. 1992. "The Ranks of Death: Secular Trends in Income and Mortality." *Health Transition Review* 2(Suppl.):29–46.

Lampang Project Staff. 1978a. "Lampang Health Development Project: A Thai Primary Health Care Approach."

———. 1978b. "Lampang Project Evaluation Progress Report No. 1. Summary Baseline Evaluation Results and Preliminary Performance Data." Lampang, Thailand. Photocopy.

———.1980. "The Lampang Health Development Project: Thailand's Fresh Approach to Rural Primary Health Care." In P. Coombs, ed., *Meeting the Basic Needs of the Rural Poor*. New York: Pergamon.

Lapham, R. J., and W. P. Mauldin. 1972. "National Family Planning Programs: Review and Evaluation." *Studies in Family Planning* 3(3).

Lapham, R. J., and G. B. Simmons, eds. 1987. *Organizing for Effective Family Planning Programs*. Washington, D.C.: National Academy Press.

Lieberman, S., Susan Stout, and A. Nyamete. 1994. "Indonesia's Health Work Force: Issues and Options." World Bank, East Asia and Pacific Region, Washington, D.C.

Long, A. F., and Stephen Harrison. 1985. *Health Services Performance: Effectiveness and Efficiency*. London and Dover, N.H.: Croom Helm.

Madhok, R. N. and International Development Association. 1974. "Manpower Requirement for Family Planning Programs." Population and Nutrition Projects Department. Washington, D.C.: International Development Association.

Makinen, Marty, and Laura Raney. 1994. "Role and Desireability of User Charges for Health Services." Draft Working Paper. Bethesda, Md.: Abt Associates.

Malison, M. D., and others. 1987. "Estimating Health Service Utilization, Immunization Coverage, and Childhood Mortality: A New Approach in Uganda." *World Health Organization Bulletin* 65(3):325–30.

Mardones, Francisco, and Barton R. Burkhalter. 1992. "Some Operational Guidelines and Issues for the Evaluation of Investments in Primary Health Care in the LAC Region." World Bank, Human Resources Division, Technical Department, Latin America and the Caribbean Region. Washington, D.C.

Mateus, Abel M. 1983. "Targeting Food Subsidies for the Needy: the Use of Cost-Benefit Analysis and Institutional Design." Working Paper 617. World Bank, Washington, D.C.

Matthias, A. R., and A. T. Green. "The Comparative Advantage of NGOs in the Health Sector— A Look at the Evidence." *World Hospitals* 39(1):10–15.

Mauldin, W. P. 1995. "Measuring Family Planning Program Sustainability." Presentation to the Task Force on Health and Family Planning Program Sustainability. USAID, Washington, D.C. Photocopy.

Mauldin, W. P., and B. Berelson. 1978. "Conditions of Fertility Decline in Developing Countries, 1965–1975." *Studies in Family Planning* 9:89–148.

Mauldin, W.P., and Robert Lapham. 1983. "Measuring Family Planning Program Effort in LDCs: 1972-1982." In Nancy Birdsall, ed., *The Effects of Family Planning Programs on Fertility in the Developing World.* Working Paper 677, Series Number 2. World Bank, Population and Development, Washington, D.C.

Mauldin, W. P., and J. A. Ross. 1991. "Family Planning Programs: Efforts and Results, 1982–1989." *Studies in Family Planning* 22(6):350–67.

McBride, Mark E., Jane T. Bertrand, R. Santiso, and J. H. Fernandez. 1987. "Cost Effectiveness of the APROFAM Program for Voluntary Surgical Contraception in Guatemala." *Evaluation Review* 11(3):300-326.

McDowell, I., and C. J. Martini. 1976. "Problems and New Directions in the Evaluation of Primary Care." *International Journal of Epidemiology* 5(3):247–50.

McKeown, Thomas. 1976. *The Modern Rise of Population.* London: Edward Arnold.

———. 1988. "The Road to Health." Presentation to a Meeting of the World Health Organization Advisory Committee on Health Research. World Health Organization Media Service. No. 131. Geneva.

Measham, Anthony. 1986. "Review of PHN Sector Work and Lending in Health, 1980–1985." , Technical Note 86-14. World Bank, Population, Health and Nutrition Department. Washington, D.C.

Mensch, Barbara, A. Fisher, Ian Askew, and A. Ajayi. 1994. "Using Situation Analysis Data to Assess the Functioning of Family Planning Clinics in Nigeria, Tanzania, and Zimbabwe." *Studies in Family Planning* 25(1):18-31.

Mills, Anne, and Michael Drummond. 1987. "Value for Money in the Health Sector: The Contribution of Primary Health Care." *Health Policy and Planning* 2(2):107–28.

Mosley, W. Henry. 1996. "Modular Questionnaire for Child Survival and Reproductive Health Program Effort. Version 1.0. Department of Population Dynamics, The Johns Hopkins University, Baltimore, Md.

Mosley, W. Henry, and S. Becker. "Demographic Models for Child Survival and Implications for Health Intervention Programs. *Health Policy and Programming* 6(3):218–33.

Mosley, W. Henry, and L. C. Chen, eds. 1984. *Child Survival: Strategies for Research. Population and Development Review.* Supplement to Vol. 10.

Murray, Christopher J. L. 1990. "Rational Approaches to priority setting in International Health. *Journal of Tropical Medicine and Hygiene* 93:303–11.

———. 1994. "Quantifying the Burden of Disease: The Technical Basis for Disability-Adjusted Life Years." *Bulletin of the World Health Organization* 72(3):429–45.

Murray, Christopher J. L., A. D. Lopez, and D. T. Jamison. 1994. "The Global Burden of Disease in 1990: Summary Results, Sensitivity Analysis and Future Directions." *Bulletin of the World Health Organization* 72(3):495–509.

Musgrove, Philip. 1989. "Fighting Malnutrition: An Evaluation of Brazilian Food and Nutrition Programs." World Bank Discussion Paper 60. Washington, D.C.

———. 1996. "Public and Private Roles in Health: Theory and Financing Patterns." Draft Working Paper. World Bank, Human Development Department, Washington, D.C.

National Conference on Evaluation of Primary Health Care Programmes and Indian Council of Medical Research. 1980. Proceedings of the Indian Council of Medical Research Conference, New Delhi, April 21–23. New Delhi: Indian Council of Medical Research.

Nepal, Central Bureau of Statistics. 1995. "Nepal Living Standards Survey: Household Questionnaire." Katmandu.

Newman, John, Laura Rawlings, and Paul Gertler. 1994. "Using Randomized Control Designs in Evaluating Social Sector Programs in Developing Countries." *The World Bank Research Observer* 9(2):181–201.

Norren, Bert Van, J. Ties Bowrma, and Esther K. Sempebwa. 1989. "Simplifying the Evaluation of Primary Health Care Programmes." *Social Science and Medicine* 28(10):1091–97.

Nottman, Dorothy, J. Halvas, and A. Rabago. "A Cost-Benefit Analysis of the Mexican Social Security Administration's Family Planning Program." *Studies in Family Planning* 17(1):1-6.

Nougtara, A., R. Sauerborn, C. Oepent, and H. J. Diesfeld. 1989. "Assessment of MCH Services Offered by Professional and Community Health Workers in the District of Solenzo, Burkina Faso. I. Utilization of MCH Services." *Journal of Tropical Pediatrics* 35(Suppl.):2–9.

Ojeda, Nestor Suarez. 1992. "Evaluation of Maternal and Child Health Services in Latin America." *World Health Forum* 13:2/3:139–42.

PAHO (Pan American Health Organization). 1986. "Health Services Utilization and Coverage: Community Based Survey in Four Caribbean Countries: Antigua/Barbuda, Dominica, St. Kitts/Nevis, and St. Lucia. Joint Country Report." Washington, D.C.

―――. "Joint Country Report: Community Based Survey on Health Services Utilization and Coverage." Antigua.

Parlato, Margaret B., and Michael N. Favin. 1992. "Progress and Problems: An Analysis of 52 AID-Assisted Projects." Washington, D.C.: American Public Health Association.

Pelletier, David L. n.d. "The Role of Information in the Planning, Management, and Evaluation of Community Nutrition Programs." Ithaca, N.Y.: Cornell University. Photocopy.

Picciotto, Robert. 1992. "Participatory Development: Myths and Dilemmas." World Bank Working Paper 930. Washington, D.C.

―――. 1994. "Visibility and Disappointment: The New Role of Development Evaluation." In Lloyd Rodwin and Donald A. Schon, eds. *Rethinking the Development Experience: Essays Provoked by the Work of A. O. Hirschman*. Washington, D.C.: The Brookings Institution.

―――. 1995. "Putting Institutional Economics to Work: From Participation to Governance." World Bank Discussion Paper 304. Washington, D.C.

Pinstrup-Andersen, Per. 1981. "Nutritional Consequences of Agricultural Projects: Conceptual Relationships and Assessment Approaches." Working Paper 456. World Bank, Washington, D.C.

Pitt, Mark M., Mark R. Rosenzweig, and Donna M. Gibbons. 1993. "Determinants and Consequences of the Placement of Government Programs in Indonesia." *World Bank Economic Review* 7:319–48.

Pole, J. D. 1973. "The Use of Outcome Measures in Health Service Planning." *International Journal of Epidemiology* 2(1).

Preston, Samuel H. 1994. "Health Indices as a Guide to Health Sector Planning: A Demographic Critique." In James N. Gribble and Samuel H. Preston, eds., *The Epidemiological Transition: Policy and Planning Implications for Developing Countries*. Washington, D.C.: National Academy Press.

Pritchett, Lant H. 1994. "Desired Fertility and the Impact of Population Policies." *Population and Development Review* 20(1):1-55.

Rashad, H., R. Gray, and T. Boerma (eds.). 1995. *Evaluation of the Impact of Health Interventions*. Liege, Belgium: International Union for the Scientific Study of Population.

Ravicz, Marisol, C. Griffin, A. Follmer, and T. Fox. 1996. "Health Policy in Eastern Africa: A Structured Approach to Resource Allocation." Green Cover. Report 14040AFR. World Bank, Africa Region, Population and Human Resources Division, Washington, D.C.

Reich, Michael R. Forthcoming. "The Political Economy of Health Transitions in the Third World." In L. C. Chen, A. Kleinman, and N. Ware, eds., *Health and Social Change in International Perspective.*

———. 1994. "Political Mapping of Health Policy: A Guide for Managing the Political Dimensions of Health Policy." School of Public Health, Harvard University, Cambridge, Mass.

———. 1995. "The Politics of Agenda Setting in International Health: Child Health Versus Adult Health in Developing Countries." *Journal of International Development* 7(3):489–502.

Reinke, W. 1980. "Health Services Program Evaluation Measures." Photocopy.

Reutlinger, Shlomo, and Marcelo Selowsky. 1975. "Undernutrition and Poverty: Magnitude and Target Group Oriented Policies." Working Paper 202. World Bank, Washington, D.C.

Reynolds, Jack, and Wayne Stinson. 1991. "Lessons Learned from Primary Health Care Programmes Funded by the AGA KHAN Foundation." Washington, D.C.: U.S. Agency for International Development.

Ridker, Ronald G. 1991. *Population and the World Bank: A Review of Activities and Impacts from Eight Case Studies*. A World Bank Operations Evaluation Study. Washington, D.C.

Rifkin, Susan B., and Gill Walt. 1986. "Why Health Improves: Defining the Issues Concerning 'Comprehensive Primary Health Care' and 'Selective Primary Health Care.'" *Social Science and Medicine* 23(6):559–66.

Robinson, Dave, and Mike Fitter. 1992. "Supportive Evaluation Methodology: A Method to Facilitate System Development." *Behavior and Information Technology* 11:151–59.

Roemer, M. I., and C. Montoya-Aguilar. 1988. "Quality Assessment and Assurance in Primary Health Care." Offset Publication 115. Geneva: World Health Organization.

Ross, John A., and E. Frankenberg. 1993. *Findings from Two Decades of Family Planning Research*. New York: The Population Council.

Rossi, Peter H., and Howard E. Freeman. 1993. *Evaluation: A Systematic Approach*. Newbury Park, Calif.: Sage.

Sauerborn, R., A. Nougtara, and H. J. Diesfeld. 1989. "Low Utilization of Community Health Workers: Results from a Household Interview Survey in Burkina Faso." *Social Science and Medicine* 29(10):1163–74.

Schieber, George J. 1995. "Preconditions for Health Reform: Experiences from the OECD Countries." *Health Policy* 32:29–293.

Scrimshaw, Nevin S., and Gary R. Gleason. 1992. *RAP, Rapid Assessment Procedures: Qualitative Methodologies for Planning and Evaluation of Health Related Programs.* Boston: International Nutrition Foundation for Developing Countries (INFDC).

Scrimshaw, Susan, and Elena Hurtado. 1987. *Rapid Assessment Procedures for Nutrition and Primary Health Care: Anthropological Approaches to Improving Programme Effectiveness.* Los Angeles: Latin American Center.

Shaw, Paul, and Charles Griffin. 1994. *Better Health in Africa. Best Practice Paper.* Washington, D.C.: World Bank.

Shaw, R. Paul, and Charles C. Griffin. 1995. *Financing Health Care in Sub-Saharan Africa Through User Fees and Insurance.* Washington, D.C.: World Bank.

Shutt, Merrill M. 1975. "Development and Evaluation of Integrated Delivery Systems." Washington, D.C.: Agency for International Development.

Sichona, Francis J., Linda Lacey, and Amy Ong Tsui. 1992. "Evaluating Family Planning Program Impact in Sub-Saharan Africa." Working Paper 92-06. Chapel Hill, N.C.: Carolina Population Center.

Simmons, George B., and D. Balk, and K. K. Faiz. 1991. "Cost Effectiveness Analysis of Family Planning Program in Rural Bangladesh: Evidence from Matlab." *Studies in Family Planning* 22(2):83-101.

Simmons, George B., and Rushikesh Maru. 1988. "The World Bank's Population Lending and Sector Review." Policy, Planning, and Research Working Paper 94. World Bank, Washington, D.C.

Simmons, Ruth, and Christopher Elias. 1993. "The Study of Client-Provider Interaction: A Review of Methodological Issues." Programs Division Working Papers 7. New York: The Population Council.

Sinding, Steven W. 1991. "Strengthening the Bank's Population Work in the Nineties." Washington, D.C.: World Bank.

Sirageldin, Ismail, and Francois Diop. 1991. "Equity and Efficiency in Health Status and Health Services Utilization: A Household Perspective." *Pakistan Development Review* 30:415–31.

Sirageldin, I., D. Salkever, and R. Osborn. 1983. *Evaluating Population Programs International Experience with Cost-Effectiveness Analysis and Cost-Benefit Analysis.* New York: St. Martin's.

Skolnik, Richard. 1987. "Nutrition Review." Photocopy. World Bank, Population, Health, and Nutrition Department, Washington, D.C.

Sloan, Frank A., ed. 1995. *Valuing Health Care: Costs, Benefits and Effectiveness of Pharmaceuticals and Other Medical Technologies*. Cambridge, U.K.: Cambridge University Press.

Smith, Gordon S. 1989. "Development of Rapid Epidemiology Assessment Methods to Evaluate Health Status and Delivery of Health Services." *International Journal of Epidemiology* 18(4)Supplement 2:S2-S14.

Solimano, Giorgia, and Poul Engerg-Pedersen. 1992. "Evaluation of UNICEF: Sector Report—Health and Nutrition." Working Paper. Evaluation under the Management of the Directors of Evaluation of AIDAB, CIDA, DANIDA and SDC.

Srinivas, Murthy A. K. and R. Parker. 1973. "New Methods for Assessing Health Care Delivery Systems." Proceedings of the 12th Annual Conference of the Indian Association for the Advancement of Medical Education, January 12–14.

Srinivasan, K. 1993. "A Critique on Contraceptive Prevalence Rate (CPR)." Paper presented at the August 1993 IUSSP General Conference, Montreal, Canada. Chapel Hill, N.C.: The Evaluation Project.

Stefanini, Angelo, and Nicola Ruck. 1992. "Managing Externally-Assisted Health Projects for Sustainability in Developing Countries." *International Journal of Health Planning and Management* 7:199–210.

St. Leger, A. S., H. Schnieden, and J. P. Walsworth-Bell. 1992. *Evaluating Health Services' Effectiveness: A Guide for Health Professionals, Service Managers, and Policy Makers*. Philadelphia: Open University Press.

Stone, Linda, and J. Gabriel Campbell. 1984. "The Use and Misuse of Surveys in International Development: An Experiment from Nepal." *Human Organization* 43(1): 27–37.

Subbarao, K. 1989. "Improving Nutrition in India: Policies and Programs and Their Impacts." World Bank Discussion Paper 49. Washington, D.C.

Tanahashi, T. 1978. "Health Service Coverage and Its Evaluation." *Bulletin of the World Health Organization* 56(2):295–303.

Tarimo, E. 1991. *Towards a Health District: Organizing and Managing District Health Systems*. Geneva: World Health Organization.

Taylor, C. 1980. "Evaluation Methodology in Primary Health Care." Paper prepared for the National Symposium on Evaluation of Primary Health Care Programs, New Delhi, India. Photocopy.

Taylor, Carl E., R. S. S. Sarma, and others. 1983. *Child and Maternal Health Services in Rural India: The Narangwal Experiment. Volume Two. Integrated Family Planning and Health Care*. Baltimore, Md.: The Johns Hopkins University Press for the World Bank.

Taylor, Carl E., R. S. S. Sarma, R. Parker, W. Reinke, and R. Faruqee. 1981. *Benefits of Integrating Family Planning with Health Services: The Narangwal Experiment.* Discussion Paper DPH8162. World Bank, Population and Human Resources Department, Washington, D.C.

Tendler, Judith. 1993. *New Lessons from Old Projects: The Workings of Rural Development in Northeast Brazil.* A World Bank Operations Evaluation Study. Washington, D.C.

Tendler, Judith, and Sara Freedheim. 1994. "Bring Hirschman Back In: A Case of Bad Government Turned Good." In Lloyd Rodwin and Donald Schon, eds., *Rethinking Development: Essays Provoked by the Work of Albert O. Hirschman.* Washington, DC: The Brookings Institution.

Tinker, Anne G. 1994. "Women's Health and Nutrition: Making a Difference." World Bank Discussion Paper 256. Washington, D.C.

Trowbridge, F., and others. 1980. "Evaluation of Nutrition Surveillance Indicators." *Pan American Health Organization Bulletin* 14(3):238–43.

Tsui, Amy. 1993a. "Improving the Effectiveness of Family Planning Programs by Improving Evaluation Capabilities." The Evaluation Project. Chapel Hill, N.C.: Carolina Population Center, University of North Carolina.

———. 1993b. "Evaluating Family Planning Program Impact: Needed Initiatives on a Persisting Question." The Evaluation Project Working Paper No. 0-08. Chapel Hill, N.C.: Carolina Population Center, University of North Carolina.

———. 1994. "A Conceptual Framework for the Evaluation of Reproductive Health." The Evauluation Project. Chapel Hill, NC: Carolina Population Center, University of North Carolina. Photocopy.

Tsui, Amy, and Luis Hernando Ochoa. 1989. "Service Proximity as a Determinant of Contraceptive Behavior: Evidence from Cross-national Studies of Survey Data" Carolina Population Center Working Paper 89-05. Chapel Hill, N.C.: University of North Carolina.

Unger, J. P. "Can Intensive Campaigns Dynamize Front Line Health Services? The Evaluation of an Immunization Campaign in Thies Health District, Senegal." *Social Science and Medicine* 32(3):249–59.

Unger, J. O., and J.R. Killingsworth. 1986. "Selective Primary Health Care: A Critical Review of Methods and Results." *Social Science and Medicine* 22:1001–13.

UNICEF. 1994. "Handbook for Multiple-Indicator Surveys." Planning and Coordination Office. New York. Photocopy.

Vaillancourt, Denise, and Stacye Brown. 1993. "Population, Health, and Nutrition: Annual Operational Review for Fiscal 1992." Working Paper Series 1152. World Bank, Population, Health, and Nutrition Department, Washington, D.C.

Valdivieso, Cecilia, and David de Ferranti. 1995. "Getting Results in the Social Sectors: An Agenda for Action." Washington, D.C.: World Bank. Photocopy.

Van Norren B., Boerma J. Ties, and E. K. N. Sempebwa. 1989. "Simplifying the Evaluation of Primary Health Care Programmes." *Social Science and Medicine* 28:1091–97.

Warford, Jeremy J. "Environment, Health, and Sustainable Development: The Role of Economic Instruments and Policies." *Bulletin of the World Health Organization* 73(3):387–95.

Wawer, Maria J., Regina McNamara, Therese McGinn, and Donald Lauro. 1991. "Family Planning Operations Research in Africa: Reviewing a Decade of Experience." *Studies in Family Planning* 22(5):279–93.

Weaving, Rachel, and Geoffrey Lamb. 1992. *Managing Policy Reform in the Real World: Asian Experience.* Washington, D.C.: EDI, World Bank.

Weiss, Michael G. 1988. "Cultural Models of Diarrheal Illness: Conceptual Framework and Review." *Social Science and Medicine* 27(1):5–16.

White, Kerr L., and R. Kohn. 1977. "Health Services: Concepts and Information for National Planning and Management: Experiences Based on the WHO/International Collaborative Study on Medical Care Utilization." World Health Organization Public Health Papers No. 67. Geneva: WHO.

Wickrama, K. A. S. and Pat M. Keith. 1990. "Use and Evaluation of Healthcare Services by Male- and Female-Headed Households in Rural Sri Lanka." *Journal of Developing Areas* 25:1–14.

Williams, Timothy, Gabriel Ojeda, and Miguel Trias. 1990. "An Evaluation of PROFAMILIA'S Female Sterilization Program in Colombia." *Studies in Family Planning* 21(5):251-264.

World Bank. n.d. "Jamaican Survey of Living Conditions Health Facilities Survey: Private Primary Health Services." Living Standards Measurement Survey. World Bank, Policy Research Department, Poverty and Human Resources Division, Washington, D.C.

———. n.d. "Pakistan Integrated Household Survey: Community-Level Questionnaires." Living Standards Measurement Survey. World Bank, Policy Research Department, Poverty and Human Resources Division, Washington, D.C.

———. 1973. "Nutrition Policy: Policy Guidelines for Bank Nutrition Activities." Sector Program Paper. Washington, D.C.

———. 1975. *Health Sector Policy Paper*. Washington, D.C.

———. 1976. "External Advisory Panel on Population. Final Report." World Bank SECM76 ("Berelson Report"). Washington, D.C.

———. 1980. *Health Sector Policy Paper*. Washington, D.C.

―――. 1982. *Malnourished People—A Policy View.* Washington, D.C.

―――. 1984a. *World Development Report 1984: Population and Development.* New York: Oxford University Press.

―――. 1984b. "Nutrition Review." Washington, D.C.

―――. 1986a. "Poverty in Latin America: The Impact of Depression." Report No. 6369. Washington, D.C.

―――. 1986b. *Poverty and Hunger.* Washington, D.C.

―――. 1987a. "Financing Health Services in Developing Countries: An Agenda for Reform." A World Bank Policy Study. Washington, D.C.

―――. 1987. "Nutrition." Washington, D.C.

―――. 1989. "Family Welfare Strategy in India: Changing the Signals." Washington, D.C.

―――. 1990. "Water Supply, Sanitation and Hygiene Education: Report of a Health Impact Study in Mirzapur, Bangladesh." Washington, D.C.

―――. 1991a. *Assistance Strategies to Reduce Poverty.* A World Bank Policy Paper. Washington, D.C.

―――. 1991b. "Population and the World Bank: A Review of Activities and Impacts from Eight Case Studies." Operations Evaluation Department. Washington, D.C.

―――. 1991c. "Tobacco Policy." Washington, D.C. Photocopy.

―――. 1992a. *Poverty Reduction: Handbook and Operational Directive.* Washington, D.C.

―――. 1992b. "Lessons from Project Experience." Southern Africa Department. Washington, D.C. Photocopy.

―――. 1992c. "Supporting Human Development: Progress and Challenges." Population and Human Resources Department. Washington, D.C.

―――. 1993. *World Development Report 1993: Investing in Health.* New York: Oxford University Press

―――. 1994a. "A New Agenda for Women's Health and Nutrition." Washington, D.C.

―――. 1994b. *Better Health in Africa: Experiences and Lessons Learned.* Washington, D.C.

―――. 1994c. "An Overview of Monitoring and Evaluation in the World Bank." Operations Evaluation Department. Washington, D.C.

———. 1994d. "Population and Development. Implications for the World Bank." Washington, D.C.

———. 1995a. *Evaluation and Development: Proceedings of the 1994 World Bank Conference.* Operations Evaluation Department. Washington, D.C.

———. 1995b. "Human Resources Development: Towards Effective Implementation." Education and Social Policy Department. Washington, D.C. Photocopy.

———. 1995c. "Investing in People. The World Bank in Action." Washington, D.C.

———. 1995d. "Sector and Project Performance Indicators for Population, Health, and Nutrition." Mimeo. World Bank, Population, Health, and Nutrition Department, Washington, D.C.

———. 1996a. *1994 Evaluation Results.* Operations Evaluation Department. Washington, D.C.

———. 1996b. "Getting Results in the Social Sectors." Human Development Department, Human Capital Vice Presidency, Washington, D.C.

———. 1996c. *Hashemite Kingdom of Jordan: Health Sector Study.* Human Resources Division, Middle East and North Africa Region, Washington, D.C.

———. 1996d. *Zimbabwe: Project Performance Audit Report.* Operations Evaluation Department, Washington, D.C.

WHO (World Health Organization). 1971. "Statistical Indicators for the Planning and Evaluation of Public Health Programmes: Fourteenth Report." Expert Committee on Health Statistics. Technical Report Series 472. Geneva.

———. 1981a. "Development of Indicators for Monitoring Progress Towards Health for All by the Year 2000." Health for All Series 4. Geneva.

———. 1981b. "Health Programme Evaluation." Health for All Series 6. Geneva.

———. 1984. "Evaluating Primary Health Care in Southeast Asia: Proceedings of a Regional Seminar." Regional Office for South-East Asia. SEARO Technical Publications 4. New Delhi.

———. 1990. *The Impact of Development Policies on Health: A Review of the Literature.* Geneva.

———. 1993. *Rapid Evaluation Method Guidelines for Maternal and Child Health, Family Planning and Other Health Services.* Division of Family Health and Division of Epidemiological Surveillance and Health Situation and Trend Assessment. Geneva.

Wouters, A. V. 1992. "Health Care Utilization Patterns in Developing Countries: Role of the Technology Environment in 'Deriving' the Demand for Health Care." *World Health Organization Bulletin* 70(3):381–89.

Yon, Ha-ch'ong, and Han'guk Kaebal Yon'guwon. 1981. *Primary Health Care in Korea: An Approach to Evaluation.* Seoul: Korea Development Institute. (Distributed outside Korea by the University Press of Hawaii.)

Zamora Zamora, Carlos Alberto. 1992. "Relationship Between Health Services Utilization and Areas of Coverage." In Kerr L. White and J. Frenk, eds., *Health Services Research: An Anthology.* PAHO Scientific Publication 534. Washington, D.C.: Pan American Health Organization.

Zimbabwe, Central Statistics Office. 1991. "Zimbabwe Service Availability Survey 1989/1990." Ministry of Finance, Economic Planning, and Development and Demographic and Health Surveys, Institute for Resource Development/Macro International, Inc. Harare, Zimbabwe, and Columbia, Md.

Zwart, Sjoerd, and Henk W. A. Voorhoeve. 1989. "Community Health Care and Hospital Attendance: A Case Study in Rural Ghana." *Social Science and Medicine* 31(7):711–18.

Zwi, Anthony, and Anne Mills. 1995. "Health Policy in Less Developed Countries: Past Trends and Future Directions" *Journal of International Development* 7(3):299–328.

Annex 1: OED Evaluated Projects and Ratings (Fiscal 1970–94), by Type, Closing Year, and Ratings

OEDID	Evaluation year	Region	Country	Name	Type	Close	Rating	Sustainability	Institutional development
A. Audits									
L0928	1982	MNA	Iran	Population project	PAR	12/31/76	Sat		
L0690	1979	LAC	Jamaica	Population project	PAR	3/31/77	Unsat		
C0437	1982	MNA	Egypt	Population project	PAR	6/30/79	Unsat		
C0468	1981	AFR	Kenya	Population project	PAR	12/31/79	Sat		
L0743	1981	LAC	Trinidad and Tobago	Population project	PAR	12/31/79	Sat		
C0312	1981	SAS	India	Population project	PAR	6/30/80	Sat		
C0238	1984	MNA	Tunisia	Population project	PAR	12/31/80	Unsat		
C0300	1985	EAP	Indonesia	Population project	PAR	12/31/81	Sat		
L0880	1985	EAP	Malaysia	Population project	PAR	12/31/81	Sat		
L1325	1985	LAC	Dominican Republic	Population and family health project	PAR	12/31/81	Sat		
C0533	1986	SAS	Bangladesh	Population project	PAR	9/30/82	Unsat		
L1035	1985	EAP	Philippines	Population project	PAR	12/31/82	Unsat		
L1284	1985	LAC	Jamaica	Second population project	PAR	12/31/82	Unsat		
L1472	1986	EAP	Indonesia	Second population project	PAR	4/30/84	Sat		
C0767	1988	EAP	Thailand	Population project	PAR	12/31/84	Sat		
L1487	1988	LAC	Colombia	Integrated nutrition improvement project	PAR	6/30/85	Sat		
L1774	1989	EAP	Korea, Republic	Population project	PAR	12/31/87	Sat	LIK	SUB
C0981	1990	SAS	India	Second population project	PAR	3/31/88	Unsat	LIK	MOD
C0923	1991	EAP	Philippines	Second Population project	PAR	6/30/88	Unsat	UNC	NEG
L2235	1990	EAP	Indonesia	Provincial health project	PAR	9/30/89	Unsat	UNC	NEG
C1653	1992	AFR	Ghana	Health and education rehabilitation	PAR	12/31/91	Sat	LIK	MOD
L2636	1993	EAP	Indonesia	Nutrition and community health project	PAR	3/31/92	Sat	LIK	SUB
C2212	1994	LAC	Honduras	First social investment fund project	PAR	3/31/94	Sat	LIK	SUB
C2401	1994	LAC	Honduras	Second social investment fund	PAR	12/31/94	Sat	LIK	SUB
B. PCRs									
L1373	1985	EAP	Indonesia	Nutrition development project	PCR	3/31/83	Sat		
L1302	1985	LAC	Brazil	Nutrition research and development	PCR	6/30/83	Unsat		
L1608	1989	EAP	Malaysia	Second population and family health	PCR	12/31/84	Unsat	UNC	NEG
L1869	1988	EAP	Indonesia	Third population project	PCR	3/31/85	Sat		
C0921	1989	SAS	Bangladesh	Second population and family health	PCR	12/31/85	Sat	LIK	MOD
C0850	1988	MNA	Egypt	Second population project	PCR	3/31/86	Unsat		

Annex 1 (Continued)

OEDID	Evaluation year	Region	Country	Name	Type	Close	Rating	Sustainability	Institutional development
L2061	1990	LAC	Brazil	Northwest region integrated development	PCR	6/30/88	Sat	UNC	NEG
C1351	1990	AFR	Malawi	Health project	PCR	12/31/88	Sat	UNC	MOD
L2005	1990	MNA	Tunisia	Health and population project	PCR	12/31/88	Sat	LIK	NEG
C1003	1990	SAS	India	Tamil Nadu integrated nutrition project	PCR	3/31/89	Sat	LIK	SUB
L2211	1993	LAC	Peru	Primary Health	PCR	6/30/89	Unsat	UNL	NEG
C1294	1990	MNA	Yemen Arab Republic	First health project	PCR	6/30/89	Unsat	UNC	MOD
C1350	1990	SAS	Pakistan	Population project	PCR	6/30/89	Unsat	UNL	MOD
L2448	1992	LAC	Brazil	National Health Policy Studies	PCR	12/31/89	Unsat	UNL	NEG
C1377	1991	MNA	Yemen, PDR	Health development project	PCR	12/31/89	Sat	UNC	MOD
C1238	1992	AFR	Kenya	Integrated Rural Health and Family	PCR	12/31/90	Sat	LIK	SUB
C1408	1992	AFR	Comoros	Health and Population	PCR	6/30/91	Unsat	UNC	NEG
C1422	1992	AFR	Mali	Health Development	PCR	9/30/91	Unsat	UNL	NEG
C1310	1993	AFR	Senegal	Rural health project	PCR	12/31/91	Sat	UNC	MOD
C1800	1993	AFR	Guinea-Bissau	Population, health and nutrition project	PCR	12/31/91	Unsat	UNL	NEG
C1472	1993	EAP	China	Rural health and medical education	PCR	12/31/91	Sat	LIK	SUB
L2413	1993	AFR	Botswana	Family health project	PCR	1/31/92	Sat	LIK	MOD
C1426	1993	SAS	India	Third population (Kerala and Karnataka)	PCR	3/31/92	Sat	UNC	MOD
L2447	1993	LAC	Brazil	Sao Paulo Basic Health Care	PCR	6/30/92	Unsat	UNC	NEG
C1649	1993	SAS	Bangladesh	Third population and family health	PCR	6/30/92	Sat	LIK	SUB
C1585	1994	AFR	Lesotho	Health and population project	PCR	12/31/92	Sat	LIK	MOD
L2529	1993	EAP	Indonesia	Fourth population project	PCR	12/31/92	Sat	LIK	MOD
L2542	1994	EAP	Indonesia	Second health (manpower development)	PCR	3/31/93	Unsat	LIK	MOD
L2503	1994	AFR	Nigeria	Sokoto health project	PCR	5/31/93	Sat	UNC	SUB
L2531	1994	MNA	Jordan	Primary health care project	PCR	5/31/93	Sat	LIK	MOD
C1768	1994	AFR	Malawi	Second family health project	PCR	6/30/93	Sat	LIK	MOD
L2611	1994	LAC	Colombia	Health services integration project	PCR	6/30/93	Unsat	UNL	MOD
L2744	1994	AFR	Zimbabwe	Family health project	PCR	9/30/93	Sat	LIK	SUB
L3306	1994	MNA	Jordan	Emergency recovery project	PCR	10/31/93	Sat	LIK	SUB
C1678	1994	AFR	Rwanda	Family health project	PCR	12/31/93	Sat	UNL	MOD
C1623	1994	SAS	India	Fourth population project	PCR	3/31/94	Sat	UNC	SUB

Source: OED Database.

Annex 2: Questionnaire on Health Care Services

OED

This is the first part of a two-part questionnaire about health care services. This part is meant to provide indicators that allow health services provided to be compared across countries. The second part, which you will fill out on the computer, will focus on management and organization and provide some feedback based on your responses.

The questions here concern your assessments of *current* service availability and utilization. (You may take mid-1996 as the reference date.) If you have strong doubts about any estimate you make or answer you give, you may add a question mark (?) after it.

Please return completed questionnaire to Susan Stout, G7-051, within one week.

Please indicate the country you are rating: _____

Name of rater: _____

Phone no.: _____

Date: _____

1. Does the country have a major, currently active program in each area below—a program recognized as a major initiative in the health sector or a distinct entity on organizational charts?

PLEASE CIRCLE THE NUMBER REPRESENTING YOUR ANSWER.

Area	Has active program	
	Yes	*No*
Immunization (EPI)	2	1
Oral rehydration therapy (ORT)	2	1
Acute respiratory infections (ARI)	2	1
Nutrition	2	1
Malaria control	2	1
Safe motherhood/maternity care	2	1
Family planning	2	1
STD/HIV	2	1
Tuberculosis control	2	1
Tobacco control	2	1
School health	2	1

2. What percent of urban and rural households have easy access to adequate public health services, and to the other general types of services listed below? (*Easy access means that reaching a source for the service—which may be either public or private—requires less than two hours, and the cost is not burdensome.*)

Service	Percent with easy access among urban households					Percent with easy access among rural households				
General medical services	<10	25	50	75	90+	<10	25	50	75	90+
Contraceptive services or supplies	<10	25	50	75	90+	<10	25	50	75	90+
Antenatal care	<10	25	50	75	90+	<10	25	50	75	90+

3.   Below is a more detailed list of services. Could you estimate the percent of households with easy access to each.

Service	Percent with easy access among urban households					Percent with easy access among rural households				
Immunization services	<10	25	50	75	90+	<10	25	50	75	90+
Oral rehydration therapy (ORT) services	<10	25	50	75	90+	<10	25	50	75	90+
Providers who can properly diagnose and treat acute respiratory infections (ARI)	<10	25	50	75	90+	<10	25	50	75	90+
Prevention and treatment of protein-energy malnutrition	<10	25	50	75	90+	<10	25	50	75	90+
Treatment for malaria	<10	25	50	75	90+	<10	25	50	75	90+
Emergency obstetric care	<10	25	50	75	90+	<10	25	50	75	90+
Abortion	<10	25	50	75	90+	<10	25	50	75	90+
Syphilis screening and treatment	<10	25	50	75	90+	<10	25	50	75	90+
Dental services	<10	25	50	75	90+	<10	25	50	75	90+

4.   Consider the typical urban health center. (Leave out the best 25% of health centers and the worst 25%.) How often would a typical center have sufficient supplies of the following commodities? Make a similar estimate for the typical rural health center.

Supplies and commodities in stock	Typical urban health center				Typical rural health center			
	At all times	Quite often	Occa-sionally	Seldom or never	At all times	Quite often	Occa-sionally	Seldom or never
Vaccines, syringes, and needles for immunization	4	3	2	1	4	3	2	1
Oral rehydration salts (ORS)	4	3	2	1	4	3	2	1
The antibiotics for acute lower-respiratory infections (ALRI) recommended in standard guidelines	4	3	2	1	4	3	2	1
Micronutrients (e.g., vitamin A, iron, iodine) as locally appropriate	4	3	2	1	4	3	2	1
Chloroquine	4	3	2	1	4	3	2	1
Tetanus toxoid vaccine	4	3	2	1	4	3	2	1
Oxytocics and anticonvulsants	4	3	2	1	4	3	2	1
Oral contraceptive pills	4	3	2	1	4	3	2	1
Condoms	4	3	2	1	4	3	2	1
Antibiotics recommended for STD treatment	4	3	2	1	4	3	2	1
Aspirin	4	3	2	1	4	3	2	1
Anthelmintics (anti-worm drugs such as mebendazole)	4	3	2	1	4	3	2	1

5.   In the typical urban or rural health center, how often you would expect to find the facilities below?

Facility	Typical urban health center				Typical rural health center			
	At all times	Quite often	Occasion-ally	Seldom or never	At all times	Quite often	Occasion-ally	Seldom or never
Clean running water	4	3	2	1	4	3	2	1
Electricity	4	3	2	1	4	3	2	1
A working refrigerator	4	3	2	1	4	3	2	1
A working X-ray machine	4	3	2	1	4	3	2	1
A sanitary toilet	4	3	2	1	4	3	2	1
A working sterilizer	4	3	2	1	4	3	2	1

6. Please indicate if each of the following statements about the typical health center is generally true or generally false in urban and rural areas.

Statement	Typical urban health center		Typical rural health center	
	True	False	True	False
The typical health center sees clients at least 30 hours a week.	2	1	2	1
The typical health center has a qualified nurse regularly and a physician at least once a week.	2	1	2	1
Staff in the typical health center have a lot of extra time on their hands.	2	1	2	1
Most patients in the typical health center are seen by a nurse or doctor within two hours of arrival.	2	1	2	1
The typical health center has enough staff to handle the daily client load.	2	1	2	1
The typical health center is visited by a supervisor, or by anyone from the district office or a higher level, at least once in six months.	2	1	2	1
The typical health center collects some fees from at least 20 percent of all clients.	2	1	2	1

7. List what you consider the three most important health problems for the population at large. In your judgment, is the health care system adequately addressing each problem?

Problem	Is problem being addressed?			
	Yes, adequately	Yes, partly	No, but receives high-level attention	No, being ignored
1st.	4	3	2	1
2nd.	4	3	2	1
3rd.	4	3	2	1

8. Are there public-sector workers whose primary task is to visit targeted, hard-to-reach women in their homes to provide child health or family planning services?

   Yes: 2   No: 1 →   *(Skip to Q. 12)*

9. What percent of the urban and the rural population is covered by such home-visiting workers?

Area	Percent of population covered by home visitors				
Urban areas	<10	25	50	75	90+
Rural areas	<10	25	50	75	90+

10. How many households is the average home-visiting worker responsible for, and how many households does he or she visit per month?

Area	Worker is responsible for:			Per month, worker visits:		
	Fewer than 500 households	500 to 2,000 households	More than 2,000 households	Fewer than 20 households	20 to 40 households	More than 40 households
Urban areas	1	2	3	1	2	3
Rural areas	1	2	3	1	2	3

11. Do any home-visiting workers provide the following health services, whether exclusively or as part of other duties?

Service	Provided by home visitors	
	Yes	No
Promotion of immunization services	2	1
Promotion of oral rehydration therapy	2	1
Diagnosis and treatment of acute respiratory infections	2	1
Prevention and treatment of malnutrition	2	1
Malaria control	2	1
Promotion of safe motherhood	2	1
Contraceptive counseling	2	1
Promotion of safe sex and STD/HIV testing	2	1

12. Consider the richest 10% of the population, and the poorest 25%. In developing countries, per capita income in the richest group is anywhere from 5 to 50 times per capita income in the poorest group. For the country you are rating, would you say this ratio is closer to 5 times or to 50 times, or somewhere in between?

Per capita income of richest 10% is *x* times per capita income of the poorest 25%

5 times	10 times	20 times	50 times

13. How easy or difficult would it be for the richest 10% and the poorest 25% to obtain the following health care services, if they were needed or desired?

Service	For richest 10%				For poorest 25%			
	Impos-sible	Very difficult	Somewhat difficult	Routine or easy	Impos-sible	Very difficult	Somewhat difficult	Routine or easy
A chest X-ray	1	2	3	4	1	2	3	4
An open-heart operation	1	2	3	4	1	2	3	4
Reliable advice about appropriate contraceptives and how to use them	1	2	3	4	1	2	3	4
Treatment for a broken arm	1	2	3	4	1	2	3	4
Chemotherapy for tuberculosis	1	2	3	4	1	2	3	4
A safe Caesarean section	1	2	3	4	1	2	3	4
Surgical repair of a hernia	1	2	3	4	1	2	3	4
Appendicitis surgery	1	2	3	4	1	2	3	4

14. Are the following health services available anywhere in the country *outside the capital city and its suburbs*?

Services	Available outside capital city and its suburbs	
	Yes	No
An EKG machine	2	1
A kidney dialysis machine	2	1
A computerized database on clinic clients	2	1
A magnetic resonance imaging (MRI) machine	2	1
An incubator for premature infants	2	1
A mammography machine	2	1

15. In comparison to government health services in various developing-country regions, where would you rank the government health services in this country?

In comparison to government health services in developing countries in:	Government health services in this country are:			
	Better than most	Above average	Below average	Worse than most
Latin America	4	3	2	1
Asia	4	3	2	1
Sub-Saharan Africa	4	3	2	1
The Middle East and North Africa	4	3	2	1

16. What proportion of the following facilities are managed by nonprofit or private agencies?

Facilities	Percent managed by nonprofits or private agencies				
Maternity centers	<10	25	50	75	90+
Hospitals with more than 20 beds	<10	25	50	75	90+

17. Please estimate the proportion of all doctors and nurses in the country who fall in each category below.

Category	Percent				
Doctors who work for the government, whether full-time or part-time	<10	25	50	75	90+
Nurses who work for the government, whether full-time or part-time	<10	25	50	75	90+
Doctors who are foreign nationals	<10	25	50	75	90+
Nurses who are foreign nationals	<10	25	50	75	90+
Doctors who are female	<10	25	50	75	90+

18. What proportion of the urban and rural population would have access to *and* would be willing to pay for a private doctor in these emergencies:

Emergency	URBAN percent with access and willing to pay a private doctor					RURAL percent with access and willing to pay a private doctor				
A child's sudden and serious illness	<10	25	50	75	90+	<10	25	50	75	90+
An accident to an adult male that could mean loss of a limb	<10	25	50	75	90+	<10	25	50	75	90+

19. Is it easier or harder for the typical *rural* resident to obtain adequate health care from any source, in comparison to the typical rural resident in other countries?

In comparison to the typical rural resident in developing countries in:	Obtaining adequate health care is:			
	Much easier	*Somewhat easier*	*Somewhat harder*	*Much harder*
Latin America	4	3	2	1
Asia	4	3	2	1
Sub-Saharan Africa	4	3	2	1
The Middle East and North Africa	4	3	2	1

Please provide us some guidance about obtaining further information.

20. Are there any accessible studies, surveys, or collections of national health statistics that would throw further light on service availability and utilization? Please indicate where they can be obtained.

Studies, surveys, or collections of national statistics	Available where?
1.	
2.	
3.	

21. Is there anyone else, in the World Bank or otherwise easily approachable, who in your estimation could give particularly reliable answers on this questionnaire?

Other possible, knowledgeable respondents	Unit or organization	Phone no. if outside Bank
1.		
2.		
3.		

Here are some final questions regarding your experience in this country.

22.   What were the dates of your most recent and your first mission to this country?

	Month	*Year*
Most recent mission:		19
First mission:		19

23.   Could you estimate the number of missions you have had to this country?   No. of missions: _____

24.   Have you authored, coauthored, or commissioned a sector report on the country's health care system or some aspect of it?

	Yes	*No*	*Title and year*
Authored or coauthored sector report	2	1	
Commissioned sector report	2	1	

25.   Your current job title   _____

Serv1.2/20Aug96

Annex 3: Questionnaire on Institutional Capacity

Evaluating Health Projects

Institutional Capacity: An interactive assessment program

The following questions are included in an interactive assessment program designed to tap opinions on the institutional capacity of the health system in a particular country. The program is available in electronic form in a Windows 3.1 compatible format, and is designed to be completed by individual respondents on diskette, and then submitted to the study team. This annex lists the questions included in the program. The program is self-scoring, enabling rapid analysis of data. The questionnaire was prepared for OED by Dr. Michael Bernhart.

This program, with only a few exceptions, will ask you to answer Yes or No [or Don't Know where that applies] to a series of questions that evaluate the sustainability of a health organization. After you have entered your answers, the sustainability of the organization will be rated on ten dimensions along with some sparse interpretation of the long term viability of the organization you have assessed.

The procedure should be fairly self-evident; place the pointer on the "button" that corresponds to your answer and click the mouse.

A   Before realistic planning can begin, information on the population to be served must be known. Does the organization or program you are assessing have reliable and current [collected within the last three years] information on the following...

A.1   The size of the under five age group
    By health district or region
    By health facility catchment area

A.2   The number of women of reproductive age
    By health district or region
    By health facility catchment area

A.3   Has the incidence of the most common diseases of children under five years of age and pregnant women been documented?
A.3.1   What is the source of that information on diseases of under fives or pregnant women?
    Survey
    Hospital and clinic records
    Mainly hospital records
    Anecdotes

A.4   Of importance in planning a maternal-child health program is information on the incidence of targeted diseases. Is the incidence of the following reliably known [reliability as used here would typically mean survey data or accurate service statistics from all health facilities]:
         Acute lower respiratory infections
         Diarrhoeal disease [are there disease specific mortality data or an indicator of severity such as hospital admissions for rehydration]
         Low birth weight [less than 2500g]
         Acute malnutrition [Gomez classification 2 or 3]
         Immunizable diseases

A.5   Is contraceptive prevalence reliably known?

B   At a minimum, planning involves using estimates of demand to project the need for supplies.

B.1   Have the diarrhoeal disease incidence data been used by the program to project demand for oral rehydration salts (ORS)?

B.2   Have the data on contraceptive prevalence and targeted increase in coverage been used by the program to project demand for contraceptives?

B.3   Have the targets for immunization been used by the program to project demand for:
         Vaccines
         Cold chain equipment
         Syringes and needles

C   Plans typically state targets or goals. Are there numerical impact targets for reducing morbidity and mortality of the under fives and pregnant women?

C.1   You answered that such targets exist. Has a date for reaching those targets, or at least many of them, been established?

C.2   Still on numerical targets or goals . . . Is there a method of monitoring progress toward them?

C.3   Of special relevance to a maternal-child health program, have quantitative and dated targets been set for:
C.3.1 ALRI mortality reduction
C.3.2 Diarrhoeal disease expressed as either a reduction in disease severity or reduction in mortality
C.3.3 Incidence of low birth rate
C.3.4 Contraceptive prevalence
C.3.5 Reduction in acute malnutrition

C.3.6 A final set of questions on targets or goal setting: Are there numerical targets for immunization coverage that are expressed in accordance with international guidelines [e.g., "80% of children will receive measles during the calendar year when between the ages of 10 and 13 months"]:
      For BCG
      For DPT
      For polio
      For measles
      For tetanus toxoid

D   Whether the program has set explicit targets or not, presumably there is interest in achieving some end. These ends may be articulated as concrete targets or as a vague interest in better health; however, both are only expressions of hope in the absence of a monitoring system, either accurate service statistics or periodic surveys, that presents to program management the degree to which health improvement goals have been achieved. Does such a system exist that produces reliable data within twelve months of the end of the planning period?

D.1 ALRI mortality reduction
D.2 Diarrhoeal disease expressed as either a reduction in disease severity or reduction in ortality
D.3 Incidence of low birth rate [less than 2500 grams]
D.4 Contraceptive prevalence
D.5 Reduction in acute malnutrition
D.6 Does this monitoring system capture immunization coverage [to include whether the vaccination occurred in accordance with international guidelines regarding the timing and number of vaccinations]:
      For BCG
      For DPT
      For polio
      For measles
      For tetanus toxoid

E   Another general, and good, indicator of the seriousness of the planning effort appears in the detail and distribution of budgets. Does the organization prepare its own annual budget?

E.1 Is the budget broken down by program [e.g., EPI, malaria, etc.]?
E.1.1 In that case, do program directors receive their budgets?

E.2 Is the budget broken down by health district or region?
E.2.1 In that case, do the directors of these areas actually receive their budgets?

E.3 Is the budget broken down by hospitals and major clinics?
E.3.1 Do the directors of these facilities receive their budgets?

E.4 Are actual financial results posted against the budget [does the accounting department record actual expenditures against budgeted expenditures]?
E.4.1 How often are the results posted, at least quarterly?
E.4.2 In that case, are the results posted monthly?

E.5   Are financial results posted at all lower levels [program, project, region, facility] for which budgets arc prepared?

E.6   Are budget performance results distributed to all managers of units or programs for which budget performance is evaluated?

You have just completed the section on planning [with questions germane to other areas embedded as well] and are one-fourth of the way through the assessment. The following questions assess the client orientation of the organization. Primary in a focus on the program's clients is knowledge of those clients. What information does the program collect, and have at its disposal, on the needs and dispositions of the target clients? Answer Yes <u>if the information is available and is known to senior program managers.</u>

A.1   Is the extent of use of ORS [oral rehydration salts] known by senior managers?

A.1.1 Beyond the extent of client use of ORS, do senior managers know the extent of client <u>acceptance</u> of ORS [they use it or they would use it if they could get it]?

A.1.2 Going one step further, is client knowledge of how to use ORS known?

A.2   Is the extent of breastfeeding known?

A.3   Is vaccination coverage known for
         BCG
         DPT
         Polio
         Measles
         Tetanus toxoid

B   A second indicator of client orientation is the existence of formal mechanisms through which clients can make their wishes and disappointments known.

B.1   Do at least half of the field supervisors contact patients in their homes or at the health facility and ask them questions about the accessibility and quality of health services?

B.2   If there are health committees at the local level, do program staff contact the majority of these committees at least quarterly for information?

B.3   When a client fails to appear for a scheduled appointment, does a staff member attempt to contact the client

B.3.1 If the missed appointment is for family planning

B.3.2 If the missed appointment is for vaccination

B.3.3 If the missed appointment is for growth monitoring of an underweight child

B.4   Is there a complaint mechanism by which patients can express their lack of satisfaction to a manager or supervisor?

C   A third indicator of a focus on clients is the existence of a <u>system</u> to monitor client satisfaction.

C.1   Are surveys of patient satisfaction with the service conducted at least every two years?

C.2   Are the following measures of factors that would affect client satisfaction taken on a biannual, or more frequent, basis?
C.2.1   Average waiting time for service in outpatient facilities
C.2.2   The number of patients per facility per day that are unable to receive outpatient service [that are turned away]
C.2.3   The percentage of patients that receive prescribed drugs and supplies [antibiotics, food supplements] at the service facility where the prescription is written

---

Obviously no quality program will be sustained if there is little attention given to preparing, motivating, and retaining staff.

A   Looking first at basic incentives . . .

A.1   Is the total package of salary and benefits roughly equivalent to what service delivery personnel could obtain in other secure employment?
A.1.1   Are staff paid on time?
A.1.2   Do staff employed in the following vertical programs receive the same compensation package [not more] as other employees at the same level within the organization?
        Vaccination
        Family planning

A.2   Do service delivery personnel advance within the program, receiving either larger salaries, more responsibility, or more status, in accordance with a formal plan?
A.2.1   Is that advancement based on either performance or seniority [that is, it is not based in the average case on caprice, connections, purchase of position, etc.]?

A.3   Will the following result, in the average case, in dismissal of a physician?
        Repeated unexcused absences from work
        Theft of program supplies
        Clear evidence of technical incompetence

A.4   Which of the following indicators are tracked by the program:
        Annual turnover rate of personnel
        Comparable private sector salaries
        Staff absenteeism

B   Skill development is obviously central to program success.

B.1   As a benchmark, indicate whether the majority of the following staff attend any formal training at least every two years.
        Physicians
        Other medical service delivery personnel
        Program managers
        Field supervisors
        Administrative/clerical personnel

B.2   Has the organization within the last two years undertaken or contracted for an evaluation of the skills needed at any technical [medical] or managerial level?

B.2.1 Has the organization offered a training course on either of the following during the past two years?

Accounting and financial analysis

Management information collection and processing

B.2.2 When such courses have been given [accounting or information collection and processing], did the program pay for at least half of the <u>direct</u> costs out of its own budget?

B.3   Is there an established training program for new health personnel in the following areas:

Breast feeding

Vaccination

Family planning

Oral rehydration therapy

Management of ALRI (acute lower respiratory infection]

Growth monitoring

Prenatal care

B.3.1 When these courses have been held, has the program paid for at least half of the <u>direct</u> costs out of its own budget?

B.3.2 Have these courses [breastfeeding, ALRI, ORT, family planning, etc.] been offered through the same training institute[s] that serve other training requirements of the organization?

C   The following two sets of questions deal with the evaluation of individual performance. In the absence of at least a rudimentary system to evaluate personnel it will be difficult to reward individual performance or correct errors.

C.1   Is there a formal periodic review mechanism for individuals in the following categories:

Physicians

Nurses

Other health care providers

Field supervisors

Administrative and clerical staff

Program managers

C.2   For those categories of personnel for whom this performance evaluation system exists, in the average case is the review performed <u>and</u> are the results shared by the reviewer with the individual who has been evaluated?

For physicians

For nurses

For health care providers other than physicians and nurses

For field supervisors

For administrative and clerical staff

For program managers

Logistics is quickly equated with management and the calibre of the logistics system is often a bellwether for other management functions. The questions in this section deal primarily with whether program management has equipped itself with the basic information and systems required to manage supplies.

A.1   Has a formulary or essential drugs list been created or adopted?

A.1.1 Are <u>any</u> drugs not on that list purchased centrally by the program?

A.2   Has a standard treatment protocol [specifying drugs and dosages] been developed or adopted for ALRI?

A.3   Do program managers have the following information available to them:

A.3.1 Draw down or use rates of
         Vaccines
         Oral rehydration salts
         Contraceptives
         The antibiotic recommended for pneumonia in children [i.e., cotrimoxazole, ampicillin, penicillin, etc.]
         Food supplements

A.3.2 Monthly stock levels of essential drugs in
         The central warehouse
         Regional warehouses
         Health facilities

A.3.3 Duration of stockouts if they occur

A.4   Are the supplies for the following maternal-child health interventions administered by the same system as other program supplies?
         Family planning
         Vaccines
         Cold chain equipment
         Oral rehydration salts

A.5   Does the host program pay at least half of the cost of the following supplies from funds not derived from donors [i.e., own budget, patient fees]?
         Contraceptives
         Oral rehydration salts
         Vaccines
         Cold chain equipment
         The antibiotic recommended for pneumonia in children [i.e., cotrimoxazole, ampicillin, etc.]
         Food supplements

B.1   Have the diarhoeal disease incidence data been used by the program [with minimal external assistance] to project demand for oral rehydration salts?

B.2   Have the data on contraceptive prevalence and targeted increase in coverage been used <u>by the program</u> [with minimal external assistance] to project demand for contraceptives?

B.3   Have the targets for immunization been used by the program to project demand for:
           vaccines
           cold chain equipment
           syringes and needles

Many would argue that field supervision is the cornerstone of any primary health care program and the following questions take up this topic.

A.1   What is the ratio of supervisors to primary care facilities to be supervised?
           Each field supervisor is responsible for
               1-10 facilities
               11-20 facilities
               Over 20 facilities
A.1.1 Are there supervisors dedicated exclusively to vertical programs?
A.1.2 For the following two vertical programs, are the salaries of the supervisors for these
       programs fully covered by funds not provided by a donor?
           Family planning
           Vaccination

A.2   To reach the facilities to be supervised what provision for transport is made for a field
       supervisor?
           Has official vehicle
           Shares offical car with others
           Is paid to use own vehicle
           Has money for public transport
           Has no transport
A.2.1 Do the supervisors for the family planning activities have the same access to
       transport,neither better nor worse,as do other field supervisors in the organization?
A.2.2 Do the supervisors for the vaccination program have the same access to transport to field
       facilities as do other field supervisors in the organization?

A.3   Do supervisors have an explicit guide to standards of care and patient counseling for
           Breast feeding
           Vaccination
           Family planning
           Management of diarrhoea
           Growth monitoring
           Management of acute lower respiratory infections
           Prenatal care

A.4   Has the supervisor been provided with or developed quantitative targets for each supervised
       facility for
           Breast feeding
           Vaccination
           Family planning
           Growth monitoring
           Prenatal care

A.5   In the average case the supervisor checks field personnel for:
       Their technical skills in maternal-child health areas
       Record keeping
       Achievement of performance targets
A.5.1 Does the supervisor, in the average case, provide performance feedback to supervisees?
A.5.2 The supervisor, on average, meets with supervisees how often?
       Monthly
       Bi-monthly
       Semi-annually
       Less often

A.6   Do field supervisors prepare reports on their visits to health facilities that are sent to program
       management?
A.6.1 Does program management provide supervisors with a written or verbal response to these
       reports?

Questions in earlier sections tapped the budget process; the following deal principally with
management's ability to determine and control costs.

A   Cost accounting. Managers cannot make prudent decisions on the cost-effectiveness of
       activities and programs without cost information.

A.1   Has the program conducted an analysis of project or activity costs within the past year [i.e.,
       cost per procedure, cost per client, cost of pharmaceuticals per client, etc.]?

A.2   Are expenses recorded in such a way that they may be assigned to projects or activities?
A.2.1 Are expenses then, in fact, assigned to programs, project, or activities?

B   Control. Can managers verify that funds have been applied to their intended uses?

B.1   Are posted expenses based on actual expenditures [usually supported by receipts, vouchers,
       etc.] and not on presumed expenses?

B.2   Are the accounts updated at least monthly?

B.3   Do the monthly, or periodic, reports show budgetary expenditures, encumbrances, and results?
B.3.1 Do the reports also show variances from budgetted amounts?

C   Managerial flexibility. A budget is a fine planning and control tool; it should not be a strait
       jacket.

C.1   Does senior management have the discretion to move limited amounts [for example, ten
       percent of the budgeted amount] from one budget category to another without seeking higher
       level approval?

C.2   Do program and facility managers have a small amount of discretionary funding to cover
       contingencies which they can spend without higher level approval?

There is no disagreement that the ability of management to resolve problems underlies its success; there is, however, disagreement over how to measure this elusive quality. The following questions concern concrete evidence of problem solving ability.

A   Creativity in problem solving. The absence of innovation in problem solving is easy to detect: endless complaining about the impossibility of resolving the problem. Innovative responses are those that go beyond conventional bureaucratic fixes and are remarked on as departures from the norm by program managers other than those who devised the responses. Can you identify at least one instance in the past 12 months when management implemented an innovative response to a problem in each of the following areas?

      Staff incentives
      External political opposition
      Internal opposition to changes
      Lack of resources

B   Recognition of problem solving capability. There is evidence that a development organization earns autonomy through demonstrated managerial competence.

B.1   Does the program prepare its own budgets?
B.1.1 Are those budgets approved without significant modification [deletion of programs, reductions in support]?

B.2   Can the organization dispose of revenues it generates [within broad guidelines]?

B.3   Can the organization establish its own structure?

C   Visible evidence of problem solving capacity is the organization's responsiveness to requests from other organizations [donors, other ministries].

C.1   When the organization receives a request for information already in hand, does it provide that information in less than one week?

C.2   Does the organization respond to requests on the status of administrative processes [i.e., status of a study, training course, etc.] within two days?

C.3   Does the organization respond to requests for decisions within two weeks?

Annex 4: Demographic, Health System, and Project Characteristics of Borrowers in HNP

Country	Population 1980 (millions)	Population 1995 (millions)	Mortality: % communic	Mortality: % non-comm	Total Fertility Rate (1995)	mortality: 0q1 (1995)	Mortality: 0q5 (1995)	1990 Pub. Health Expend (% GDP)	1990 Priv. Health Expend (% GDP)	1990 Health Expend (1990 US$ per cap)	Proj. Status	Major Sector	Project Name	FY	L/C No.	L/C $
AFRICA			68.2	23.9												
ANGOLA	7.1	11			6.9	118	184				Active	HE	HEALTH	1993	C24900	19900000
BENIN	3.4	5.4			6.9	83	161	1.1	1.6	19	Active	HE	HEALTH SERVICES DEV	1989	C20310	18600000
											Active	HP	POPULATION AND HEALT	1995	C27340	27800000
BOTSWANA		1.5			4.7			3.8	1.3	139	Completed	HP	FAMILY HEALTH	1984	L24130	11000000
BURKINA FASO	6.1	10.3			6.3	126	189	0.8	1.5	7	Active	HE	HEALTH I	1985	C16070	26600000
											Active	HE	HEALTH/NUTRITION	1994	C25950	29200000
											Active	HE	POPULATION/AIDS CONT	1994	C26190	26300000
BURUNDI	4.1	6.4			6.5	99	146	1.4	1.6	30	Completed	HE	HEALTH/POP.I	1988	C18620	14000000
											Active	HY	SOCIAL ACTION	1993	C24940	10400000
											Active	HE	HEALTH/POPULATION II	1995	C27310	21300000
CAMEROON	8.4	13.2			5.5	59	113	0.7	1.6	27	Completed	HY	SDA/HUMAN RESOURCES	1990	L32060	21500000
											Active	HY	HLTH/FERT/NUTRITION	1995	C26840	43000000
CHAD	4.5	6.4			5.7	117	175	1.5	1.5	18	Active	HY	SOCIAL DEV PRG	1990	C21560	23200000
											Active	HE	HEALTH & SAFE MOTHER	1994	C26260	18500000
											Active	HP	POP. & AIDS CO	1995	C26920	20400000
COMOROS		0.6			6.8	84	114	2.5	1.6	28	Completed	HP	POPULATION & HEALTH	1984	C14080	2850000
											Active	HP	POP & HUMAN RESOURCES	1994	C25530	13000000
COTE DIVOIRE	8.3	14.3			7.1	90	138	1.6	1.6	28	Completed	HE	HEALTH I	1986	L26190	22200000
											Active	HE	HEALTH IMPROVEMENT PROJECT	1992	C23480	5500000
EQ. GUINEA		0.4			5.7	112	171	2.8	1.5	4	Active	HP	FAMILY HEALTH	1988	C19130	33000000
ETHIOPIA	31.1	55.1			6.8	113	174	1.6	1.6	22	Active	HP	POP/HEALTH	1987	C17600	5600000
GAMBIA		1.2			5.4	127	193	2.1	1.6		Active	HY	WOMEN IN DEVELOPMENT	1990	C21410	7000000
GHANA	11.7	17.5			5.7	77	113	1.2	1.8	15	Completed	HE	HEALTH&EDUC.REHAB.	1986	C16530	15000000
											Active	HE	HEALTH & POP II	1991	C21930	27000000
GUINEA	5.4	6.7			6.8	129	200	1.6	1.6	17	Active	HE	POP/HEALTH	1988	C18370	19700000
											Active	HE	HEALTH/NUT.SCTR.	1994	C25740	24600000
GUINEA-BISSAU		1.1			5.6	135	207	2.6	1.5	16	Completed	HE	PHN	1987	C18000	4200000
KENYA	15.9	28.3			6	68	107	1.7	1.6	16	Completed	HP	POPULATION I	1974	C04680	8800000
											Completed	HP	POPULATION II	1982	C12380	12000000
											Active	HP	POPULATION III	1988	C19040	23000000
											Active	HP	POPULATION IV	1990	C21100	12200000
											Active	HE	HEALTH REHABILITATION	1992	C23100	35000000
											Active	HE	SEXUALLY TRANSMITTED	1995	C26860	40000000
LESOTHO	1.3							3.2	2.2	26	Completed	HE	HEALTH/POP.	1985	C15850	3500000
											Active	HE	HEALTH/POP.II	1990	C20590	12100000
MADAGASCAR	8.7	14.8			5.9	93	125	0.7	1.3	7	Active	HE	NAT HEALTH SECTOR	1991	C22510	31000000
											Active	HN	FOOD SECURITY & NUTRITION	1993	C24740	21300000
MALAWI	6.1	11.1			6.9	139	215	1.7	2.1	11	Completed	HE	HEALTH-NUTRITION	1983	C13510	6800000
											Completed	HE	SECOND FAMILY HEALTH	1987	C17680	11000000
											Active	HP	PHN SECTOR CREDIT	1991	C22200	55500000
MALI	7	10.8			6.9	154	188	1.3	2.4	15	Completed	HE	HEALTH DEVT PROJECT	1984	C14220	16700000
											Active	HE	HEALTH/POPULATION/RURAL W/S	1991	C22170	26600000
MAURITANIA	1.5	2.3			5.2	96	145	1.1	1.6	18	Active	HE	POP HEALTH	1992	C23110	15700000
MOZAMBIQUE	12.1	16			6.3	143	179	1.2	1.5	5	Active	HE	HEALTH & NUTRITION	1989	C19890	27000000
											Active	HE	FOOD SECURITY	1993	C24870	6300000
NIGER	5.3	9.1			7.3	119	186	1.7	1.6	16	Active	HE	HEALTH	1986	C16680	27800000
											Active	HP	POPULATION	1992	C23600	17600000
NIGERIA	84.7	111.7			6.2	81	149	1	1.6	10	Completed	HE	SOKOTO HEALTH PROJEC	1985	L25030	34000000
											Active	HE	IMO HEALTH & POPULAT	1989	L30340	27600000
											Active	HE	NAT.ESS.DRUGS	1990	L31250	68100000
											Active	HP	POPULATION	1991	C22380	78500000
											Active	HP	HEALTH FUND	1991	L33260	70000000
RWANDA	5.2	8			6.3	108	162	0.5	1.6	10	Completed	HE	FAMILY HEALTH	1986	C16780	10800000
											Active	HP	POPULATION	1991	C22720	19600000
											Active	HY	FOOD SEC & SOCIAL ACTION PROJ	1992	C23880	19100000
SAO TOME & P								2.7	1.6	38	Active	HE	HEALTH & EDUCATION	1992	C23430	11400000
SENEGAL	5.7	8.3			5.8	65	160	1.7	1.7	29	Completed	HP	RURAL HEALTH	1983	C13100	15000000
											Active	HP	HUMAN RES I (POP/HEA	1991	C22550	35000000

Country	Population 1980 (millions)	Population 1995 (millions)	Mortality: % communic	Mortality: % non-comm	Total Fertility Rate (1995)	mortality: 0q1 (1995)	Mortality: 0q5 (1995)	1990 Pub. Health Expend (% GDP)	1990 Priv. Health Expend (% GDP)	1990 Health Expend (1990 US$ per cap)	Proj. Status	Major Sector	Project Name	FY	L/C No.	L/C $
SIERRA LEONE	3.5	4.5									Active	HN	COMM NUTRITION	1995	C27230	18200000
TANZANIA	18.7	29.7			6.3	160	246	0.5	0.8	4	Active	HE	POP/HEALTH	1986	C16950	5300000
TOGO	2.5	4.1			5.7	83	128	0.7	1.5		Active	HE	HEALTH & NUTRITION	1990	C20980	4760000
UGANDA	12.6	21.3			6.3	81	121	1.7	1.6	18	Active	HE	POPULATION/HEALTH AD	1991	C22110	14200000
					7	113	174	0.5	1.8	8	Active	HE	FIRST HEALTH	1988	C19340	42500000
											Active	HY	POVERTY & SOC COSTS	1990	C20880	28000000
											Active	HE	SEXUAL TRANS.IN	1994	C26030	50000000
ZAIRE	28.3	29.7			6.5	89	133	0.2	1.5	5	Active	HP	DISTRICT HEALTH	1995	C26790	45000000
											Completed	HE	AIDS	1989	C19530	8100000
ZAMBIA	5.8	9.5			5.7	102	141	2.1	1	17	Active	HY	SOC SEC PROJECT	1991	C21960	20000000
											Active	HP	SOCIAL RECOVERY PROJ	1991	C22730	20000000
											Active	HE	SOCIAL RECOVERY II	1995	C27550	30000000
ZIMBABWE	7.4	11.3			4.8	66	104	2.5	3	39	Active	HE	HEALTH SECTOR	1995	C26600	56000000
											Completed	HE	FAMILY HEALTH	1987	L27440	10000000
											Active	HE	FAMILY HLTH.II	1991	L33390	25000000
											Active	HE	STI	1993	C25160	64500000
											Active	HE	IODINE DEF. DISORDER	1995	C27560	27000000
EAST ASIA			41.8	49.6												
CHINA	976.7	1221.1	15.1	73.4	2	41	44	2.1	1.4	11	Completed	HE	RURAL HEALTH/MED ED.	1984	C14720	85000000
											Active	HE	HEALTH II	1986	C17130	80000000
											Active	HE	REG.HEALTH SERVICES (HLTH III)	1989	C20090	52000000
											Active	HE	INFECTIOUS DISEASES	1992	C23170	129600000
											Active	HE	RUR HEALTH MANPOWER DEV	1994	C25390	110000000
											Active	HE	MATERNAL CHILD HEALT	1995	C26550	90000000
INDONESIA	146.6	197.6			2.8	52	65	0.5	1.3	12	Completed	HP	POPULATION I	1972	C03000	13200000
											Completed	HP	POP. II	1977	L14725	24500000
											Completed	HN	NUTRITION	1977	L13735	13000000
											Completed	HP	POP. III	1980	L18695	35000000
											Completed	HE	HEALTH I	1983	L22350	27000000
											Completed	HP	POPULATION IV	1985	L25290	46000000
											Completed	HE	HEALTH MANPOWER	1985	L25420	39000000
											Completed	HN	NUTRITION/COM.HEALTH	1986	L26360	33400000
											Active	HE	THIRD HEALTH PROJECT	1989	L30420	43500000
											Active	HE	POPULATION V	1991	L32980	104000000
											Active	HE	THIRD COMM HEALTH & NUTRITION	1993	L35500	93500000
KOREA	38.2	45			1.8	10	13	2.7	3.9	265	Active	HE	HEALTH IV:IMPR HEALT	1995	L39050	88000000
											Completed	HP	POPULATION I	1980	L17745	30000000
											Completed	HE	HEALTH TECH I	1991	L33300	60000000
LAO, P.D.R.	3.4	4.9			6.4	91	148	0.4	1.5	5	Active	HE	HEALTH II	1993	L35160	30000000
MALAYSIA	13.9	20.1			3.4	12	23	1.3	1.7	71	Active	HE	HEALTH SYS. REF. & M	1995	C26740	19200000
											Completed	HP	POPULATION	1973	L08800	5000000
											Completed	HP	POP. II	1979	L16085	17000000
PAPUA NEW G.	3	4.3			4.8	65	84	2.6	1.6	37	Active	HE	HEALTH	1994	L36820	50000000
PHILIPPINES	49	67.6			3.8	39	48	1	1	16	Active	HP	POPULATION PROJECT	1993	L35910	6900000
											Completed	HP	POPULATION	1975	L10355	25000000
											Completed	HP	POPULAT. II	1979	C09230	40000000
											Active	HE	HEALTH DEVELOPMENT	1989	L30990	70100000
											Active	HE	URB HEALTH & NUTRITI	1993	C25060	40000000
THAILAND	47	58.8			2.1	35	43	1	3.9	72	Active	HE	WOMENS HEALTH & SAFE	1995	L38520	18000000
											Completed	HP	POPULATION I	1978	C07670	33100000
MIDDLE EAST			46.2	44.8												
ALGERIA	18.9	27.9			3.6	49	56	5.3	1.6	149	Completed	HE	PILOT PUBLIC HEALTH	1991	L32990	16000000
EGYPT	39.8	62.9			3.7	61	73	0.8	1.6	28	Completed	HP	POPULATION	1974	C04370	5000000
											Completed	HP	POPULATION II	1979	C08500	25000000
											Active	HY	EMERGENCY SOCIAL FUN	1991	C22760	140000000
IRAN	38.8	67.3			4.8	32	62	1.4	1.1	244	Active	HE	SCHISTOSOMIASIS CONT	1992	C24030	26840000
											Completed	HP	POPULATION	1973	L09280	16500000
JORDAN	3.2	5.4			5.4	33	41	1.4	2	55	Active	HE	HEALTH AND FAMILY PL	1993	L35840	141400000
											Completed	HE	HEALTH	1985	L25310	13500000

Country	Population 1980 (millions)	Population 1995 (millions)	Mortality: % communic	Mortality: % non-comm	Total Fertility Rate (1995)	mortality: 0q1 (1995)	Mortality: 0q5 (1995)	1990 Pub. Health Expend (% GDP)	1990 Priv. Health Expend (% GDP)	1990 Health Expend (1990 US$ per cap)	Proj. Status	Major Sector	Project Name	FY	L/C No.	L/C $
LEBANON	2.7	3			2.9	31	37				Active	HE	HEALTH II	1993	L35740	20000000
MOROCCO	20.2	27			3.4	62	80	0.9	1.6	26	Active	HE	HEALTH PROJECT	1995	L38290	35700000
												HE	HEALTH DEVELOPMENT	1985	L25720	28400000
											Active	HE	HEALTH SECTOR INVEST	1990	L31710	104000000
OMAN		2.2			6.9	27	34	2.5	1.7	209	Active	HE	HEALTH	1987	L28070	13300000
TUNISIA	6.4	8.9			3	40	51	3.1	1.6	76	Completed	HP	POPULATION	1971	C02380	9600761.8
											Completed	HP	HEALTH & POPULATION	1981	L20050	12500000
											Active	HE	HOSPITAL MGT. & FIN.	1991	L33080	30000000
											Active	HE	POPULATION & FAMILY	1991	L33070	26000000
YEMEN	7	14.5			7.4	114	159	1.1	1.7	20	Completed	HE	HEALTH I	1983	C12940	10500000
											Completed	HN	HEALTH DEV.I	1983	C13770	7600000
											Active	HN	HEALTH II	1989	C19720	4500000
											Active	HE	HEALTH II	1990	C21510	15000000
											Active	HP	EMERGENCY RECOVERY C	1991	C22580	33000000
											Active	HY	FAMILY HEALTH	1993	C25250	26600000
LATIN AMERICA/CARIBBEAN			32.3	57.9												
ARGENTINA	27.7	34.6			2.7	23	26	2.5	1.7	137	Active	HP	MTNAL CHILD HLTH & NUTRI	1994	L36430	100000000
											Active	HE	PROVCL HLTH SCTR DEV	1996	L39310	101400000
BOLIVIA	5.6	7.4			4.6	70	91	1.6	1.6	25	Active	HY	SOC INV FUND	1990	C21270	20000000
											Active	HE	INTEGRATED HLTH DEV	1990	C20920	20000000
BRAZIL	118.7	161.8			2.8	56	70	2.8	1.4	146	Completed	HN	NUTRITION I	1976	L13020	19000000
											Completed	HP	NW DEVT I - HEALTH	1982	L20610	13000000
											Completed	HP	SAO PAULO HEALTH	1984	L24480	2000000
											Completed	HP	SAO PAULO HEALTH	1984	L24470	55500000
											Completed	HP	NE BASIC HLTH SRV I	1986	L26990	59500000
											Active	HE	NE ENDEMIC DIS. CTL	1988	L29310	109000000
											Active	HE	AMAZON BASIN MALARIA	1989	L30720	99000000
											Active	HE	NE BASIC HLTH SRV II	1990	L31350	267000000
											Active	HE	AIDS CONTROL	1994	L36590	160000000
CHILE	11.1	14.3			2.5	15	17	3.3	1.4	100	Active	HE	T.A. & RHB PROJ	1992	L34270	27000000
											Active	HE	HEALTH SECTOR	1993	L35270	90000000
COLOMBIA	26.7	35.1			2.6	36	41	1.8	2.2	51	Completed	HN	NUTRITION	1978	L14870	25000000
											Completed	HE	PUBLIC HEALTH	1986	L26110	36500000
											Active	HE	COMM CHILD CARE & NUTRI	1990	L32010	24000000
											Active	HN	MUNICIPAL HEALTH SERVICES	1993	L36150	50000000
COSTA RICA	2.2	3.4			3	13	15	4.8	1.6	132	Active	HE	HEALTH SECTOR REFORM	1994	L36540	22000000
DOMINICAN R.	5.4	7.8			2.9	37	48	2	1.6	38	Completed	HP	FAMILY WELFARE	1977	L13250	5000000
											Active	HE	SOC DEVT II/HEALTH&NUTRITION	1993	L35100	70000000
ECUADOR	8	11.5			3.3	47	58	2.3	1.6	44	Active	HE	SOC SEC HLTH	1991	L33480	26000000
EL SALVADOR	4.5	5.8			3.8	42	65	1.7	3.3	58	Active	HE	SOCIAL INV FUND	1993	L35340	20000000
GUATEMALA	7.3	10.6			5.1	44	69	1.6	1.6	27	Active	HE	HEALTH,NUTRITION & SANITATION	1992	C23580	10300000
GUYANA	5	0.8			2.4	45	63	4.2	1.6	42	Active	HP	HLTH & POPULATN	1990	C20850	28200000
HAITI	5	7.2			4.7	82	107	1.8	3.8	27	Active	HP	ECON & SOC FUND	1991	C22050	11300000
HONDURAS	3.7	5.7			4.6	39	52	2.6	1.6	52	Completed	HE	SOCIAL FUND	1991	C22120	20000000
											Active	HE	SOC INV FUND II	1992	C24010	10200000
											Active	HN	NUTRITION/HLTH	1993	C24520	25000000
JAMAICA	2.2	2.4			2.2	13	21	2.9	1.7	83	Completed	HP	FAMILY PLANNING	1970	L06900	20000000
											Completed	HP	POPULATION II&NUTRIT	1976	L12840	6800000
											Active	HE	POPULATN & HLTH I	1987	L28510	10000000
											Active	HP	SOC SCTR INVT LN	1990	L31110	30000000
MEXICO	69.8	93.7			3	34	41	1.6	1.6	89	Active	HE	BASIC HEALTH	1991	L32720	180000000
NICARAGUA	2.6	4.4			4.8	48	69	4.9	1.9	34	Active	HE	SOC INV FUND	1993	C24340	25000000
											Active	HP	HEALTH SECTOR PROJECT	1994	C25560	15000000
PANAMA	17.4	2.6			2.8	23	29	5.2	1.7	142	Active	HE	RURAL HEALTH	1995	L38410	25000000
PERU	17.4	23.8			3.3	61	73	1.8	1.3	61	Completed	HE	HEALTH	1983	L22110	33500000
											Active	HP	BASIC HLTH/NUTRITION	1994	L37010	34000000
TRINIDAD & T	1.2	1.3			2.3	17	17	2.8	1.7	180	Completed	HP	FAMILY PLANNING	1971	L07430	3000000
URUGUAY	2.9	3.2			2.3	18	21	2.5	2.1	123	Active	HE	HLTH SCTR DEVT	1995	L38550	15600000
VENEZUELA	14.9	21.9			3.1	22	25	2	1.6	88	Active	HN	SOCIAL DEVT	1991	L32700	105000000
											Active	HE	ENDEMIC DISEASE CONTROL	1993	L35380	94000000

Country	Population 1980 (millions)	Population 1995 (millions)	Mortality: % communic	Mortality: % non-comm	Total Fertility Rate (1995)	mortality: 0q1 (1995)	Mortality: 0q5 (1995)	1990 Pub. Health Expend (% GDP)	1990 Priv. Health Expend (% GDP)	1990 Health Expend (1990 US$ per cap)	Proj. Status	Major Sector	Project Name	FY	L/C No.	L/C $
EASTERN EUROPE																
ALBANIA	2.7	3.4	3.6	86.8							Active	HE	HEALTH SERVICE REFOR	1995	L38230	54000000
					2.8	28	39	3.4	0.6	26	Active	HE	HEALTH SERVICES REHA	1995	C26590	12400000
CROATIA		4.5			1.7	8	17				Active	HE	HEALTH PROJECT	1995	L38430	40000000
ESTONIA		1.5			1.6	16	19	1.9	1.7	228	Active	HE	HEALTH	1995	L38350	18000000
HUNGARY	10.8	10.1			1.7	15	17	5	0.9	185	Active	HE	HEALTH SERVICES AND	1993	L35970	91000000
POLAND	35.8	38.4			1.9	13	18	4.1	1	84	Active	HE	HEALTH	1992	L34660	130000000
ROMANIA	22.2	22.8			1.5	22	29	2.4	1.5	58	Active	HE	HEALTH SERVICES REHA	1992	L34090	150000000
TURKEY	44.9	61.9			3.2	58	68	1.4	2.5	76	Active	HE	HEALTH I	1989	L30570	75000000
											Active	HE	HEALTH II	1995	L38020	150000000
SOUTH ASIA																
BANGLADESH	88.5	120.4	41.8	49.6	4.1	102	148	0.8	1.8	6	Completed	HP	POPULATION I	1975	C05330	15000000
											Completed	HP	POPULATION II	1979	C09210	32000000
											Completed	HP	POPULATION III	1986	C16490	78000000
											Active	HE	POP. & HEALTH IV	1991	C22590	180000000
											Active	HN	NUTRITION	1995	C27350	59800000
INDIA	673.2	935.7	43.3	50.2	3.6	77	102	1.2	4.7	21	Completed	HP	POPULATION	1972	C03120	21200000
											Completed	HP	POPULATION II	1980	C09810	46000000
											Completed	HN	NUTRITION	1980	C10030	32000000
											Completed	HP	POPULATION III	1984	C14260	70000000
											Completed	HE	W. BENGAL POPULATION	1986	C16230	51000000
											Active	HP	BOMBAY & MADRAS POP.	1988	C19310	57000000
											Active	HP	FAMILY WELFARE TRG (	1989	C19310	124600000
											Active	HN	SECOND TN NUTRITION	1990	C21580	95800000
											Active	HP	POP. TRG (VII)	1990	C21330	96000000
											Active	HN	ICDS I (ORIS & ANDHR	1991	C21730	202000000
											Active	HE	AIDS PREVENTION AND	1992	C23500	84000000
											Active	HP	POPULATION VIII	1992	C23940	79000000
											Active	HE	HEALTH I (MCH)	1992	C23940	214500000
											Active	HP	ICDS II (BIHAR & MP)	1993	C24700	194000000
											Completed	HE	NATL LEPROSY ELIMINA	1993	C25280	85000000
											Active	HP	SOCIAL SAFETY NETS	1993	C24480	500000000
											Active	HE	POPULATION IX	1994	C26300	88600000
											Active	HE	BLINDNESS CONTROL	1994	C26110	117800000
											Active	HE	AP 1ST REF. HEALTH S	1995	C26630	133000000
NEPAL	14.6	21.9			5.2	93	126	1	2.3	7	Active	HP	POPULATION & HEALTH	1994	C26000	267000000
PAKISTAN	82.2	140.5			5.9	82	107	1.7	1.6	12	Completed	HP	POPULATION	1983	C13500	18000000
											Active	HE	FAMILY HEALTH	1991	C22400	45000000
											Active	HE	FAMILY HEALTH II	1993	C24640	48000000
											Active	HP	POPULATION WELFARE P	1995	C26880	65100000
SRI LANKA		18.4			2.4	16	20	1.5	1.9	18	Active	HE	HEALTH & POPULATION	1988	C19030	17500000
											Active	HP	POVERTY ALLEVIATION	1991	C22310	57500000

ProjectNumber: _____   **L/C No.:** _____

Country: _____   **Region:** _____   **OED ID:** _____

ProjectName: _____   **DateCoded:** _____

CoderInitials: _____   **Year:** _____

Economic and Epidemiological Analysis

1. Did the SAR justify this project among the universe of possible interventions in the sector, as well as in related sectors? (**SARJustification**)

    0: not at all

    1: considered/discussed the costs and effectiveness of this intervention

    2: compared costs and effectiveness of this intervention to others in the sector

    3: compared costs and effectiveness of this intervention to others in the sector, as well as to interventions in other sectors that might address the same needs

2. Did the SAR consider demand for the proposed interventions? (**SARDemand**)

    0: not at all

    1: Considered alternatives available to households

    Included evidence concerning demand for proposed services

      2: for some components   3: for most components

    Made rough estimates of net effect of proposed intervention

      4: for some components   5: for most components

3. How much beneficiary involvement was there in project design? (**BenefInvolvement**)

    0: not mentioned

    1: design responds to perceived consumer concerns

    2: consumers interviewed or surveyed by Bank or others

    3: consumers given decision making power

4. Did the SAR justify public sector involvement for the projects in question? (**PubSectInvolvement**)

    0: not at all

    1: mentioned market failures, public goods, or externalities

    2: identified market failures in the country and sector in question

    3: described and weighed both market failure and potential government failure

5. Did the SAR present an account of the future of the HNP sector in the country if the project were not implemented? (**Futurew/oImplementation**)

    0: not at all

    1: assumed without argument that current trends will continue

    2: estimated output or outcome data in absence of project

    3: compared estimates of both outputs and outcomes both with and without the project

6. Did the SAR estimate the supply of health inputs in the absence of the proposed project? (**SupplyHealthInputs**)

    0: not at all

    1: provided data on public and private providers

    2: developed hypotheses concerning concerning relative magnitudes of supply elasticities, e.g., potential crowding out or "in"

    3: considered both crowding out ("in") and potential effect of public-private competition

7. Did the SAR analyze the fiscal impact of the proposed project? (**FiscalImpact**)
> 0: not at all
> 1: estimated recurrent burden of project for government
> 2: discussed recurrent burden in context of total tax burden and public debt
> 3: also analyzed impact of expenditures on labor markets

8. If project involved health facility construction, what criteria was used to determine location? (**LocationCriteria**)
> 0: not discussed
> 1: average population per facility
> 2: statistics identifying underserved population, including private providers
> 3: all of the above, including consultation with local authorities and beneficiaries

9. Did the SAR identify the health needs of the country? (**HealthNeeds**)
> 0: not at all
> 1: described the country's epidemiological profile
> 2: ranked the needs on the basis of analyses of burden of disease or other method
> 3: the ranking method also included input from consumers on relative importance

10. Did the SAR include a cost-benefit, cost-utility, or cost-effectiveness analysis? (**CBCUCEAnalysis**)
> 0: not at all
> 1: claimed that the project would be cost-effective
> 2: included data on the unit costs of the interventions
> 3: included a formal CB, CU, or CE analysis

11. Did the SAR include a risk analysis for the proposed project? (**RiskAnalysis**)
> 0: not at all
> 1: described institutional, economic, environmental, or other risks
> 2: assigned weights or ranks to the various risks
> 3: included a formal risk analysis

12. Did the SAR discuss strategies to benefit the poor? (**BenefitPoor**)
> 0: not at all
> 1: asserted that the poor will benefit
> 2: discussed alternative strategies for increasing benefits to the poor, or for increasing the numbers of poor who will benefit
> 3: weighed the poverty benefits and administrative costs of alternative targeting strategies

13. Did the SAR discuss user fees/cost recovery? (check all that apply)
> - no mention (**UserFeesNoMention**)
> - a system of user fees exists in the country (**UserFeesExists**)
> - plans in project to study fees (consumers' willingness to pay/private out-of-pocket expenses on health) (**UserFeesStudyPlans**)
> - plans by project/government to introduce or strengthen user fees (may include self-financing health insurance, e.g., pre-payment schemes) (**UserFeesPlansIntroduce**)

For NA: Leave Blank

Institutional and political analysis

14. What was the level of national (or, for federal countries, provincial) government involvement in project design or preparation? (**NatlGovtInvolvement**)
    0: not mentioned
    1: government officials interviewed/consulted
    2: government officials designed some components of project
    3: government designed most of project

15. What was the level of provincial (or, for federal countries, municipal) government involvement in project design or preparation? (**ProvGovtInvolvement**)
    0: not mentioned
    1: government officials interviewed/consulted
    2: government officials designed some components of project
    3: government designed most of project

16. What evidence did the SAR provide of government commitment? (**GovtCommitment**)
    0: not mentioned
    1: asserted that government is committed
    2: cited government's actions to facilitate the project prior to appraisal
    3: cited government's passage of a law to facilitate the project prior to appraisal

17. Did the SAR analyze the institutional obstacles to the project? (**InstitutionalObstacles**)
    0: not at all
    1: discussed commitment to project
    2: analyzed incentive structures of central government officials, local government officials, bureaucrats, or service providers
    3: analyzed incentive structures of all of the above

18. Did the SAR consider the potential negative consequences of the project on borrower institutions? (**NegativeConsequences**)
    0: no
    1: yes

19. If the project sought to decentralize authority for public health care, did the SAR address incentives at the local or regional levels? (**DecentralizIncentives**)
    0: not at all
    1: addressed the legal or political independence of municipal or provincial leaders from center
    2: addressed local leaders' independence from center as well their relationships to service providers
    3: addressed potential conflicts between consumer demands on local leaders and political demands from other groups

20. Did the SAR include an analysis of the political economy of the sector? (**PoliticalEconomy**)
    0: not at all
    1: asserted potential resistance on the part of bureaucrats, providers, suppliers or others
    2: analyzed the nature of the interest group influence on the executive, legislature, or other government body
    3: proposed strategies to counter influence and resistance

For NA: Leave Blank

21. For which of the following dimensions did the SAR assess the implementing agencies?
    _ regulatory and legal framework (**AgenciesRegulatory**)
    _ targets or goals (for health, utilization, institutional performance) (**AgenciesTargets**)
    _ expenditure and financial controls (**AgenciesControls**)
    _ planning and budgeting systems (**AgenciesSystems**)
    _ consumer and service information (**AgenciesInformation**)
    _ monitoring (health, consumer satisfaction, employees) (**AgenciesMonitoring**)
    _ staff development (**AgenciesStaff**)
    _ logistics (**AgenciesLogistics**)
    _ incentives (for government officials and providers) (**AgenciesIncentives**)

Performance indicators and evaluation

22. If the project sought to improve health status, did the SAR present indicators to assess health status outcomes? (**StatusOutcomes**)
    0: not at all
    1: mentioned indicators related to the project
    2: provided baseline indicators and projected values after successful implementation
    3: projected values based on analysis of causal links between project components and indicators

23. If the project sought to improve health status, did the SAR present indicators to assess intermediate outcomes (e.g., utilization, vaccination)? (**IntermediateOutcomes**)
    0: not at all
    1: mentioned indicators related to the project
    2: provided baseline indicators and projected values after successful implementation
    3: projected values based on analysis of causal links between project components and indicators

24. If the project sought to improve health status, did the SAR present indicators to assess project outputs (numbers of doctors trained, clinics built, etc.)? (**ProjectOutputs**)
    0: no
    1: some components
    2: most components

25. If the project sought to improve system performance, did the SAR present indicators to assess system performance (efficiency, equity, etc.)? (**SystemPerformance**)
    0: no
    1: some components
    2: most components

26. Did project propose to collect data on who actually benefited? (**DataCollectionBenef**)
    0: no
    1: some components
    2: most components

For NA: Leave Blank

27. Did the SAR discuss data collection regarding outcomes and its management? (**DataCollectionOutcomes**)
>   0: not at all
>   1: plans to develop and collect data regarding outcomes/outputs
>   2: specified unit and described methodology
>   3: specified unit, methodology, and discussed feedback of data into project

28. Did the SAR analyze borrower incentives and capacity for collecting monitoring and evaluation data? (**BorrIncentivesM&E**)
>   0: no
>   1: yes

29. Did the SAR plan to obtain feedback from beneficiaries? (**BenefFeedback**)
>   0: no mention
>   1: feedback through project staff
>   2: feedback through surveys
>   3: feedback using participatory evaluation methods

30. If the project attempted to increase demand for HNP interventions (IEC), did the SAR include: _ none (**DemandIECNone**)
>   _ market research to evaluate IEC materials (**DemandIECMktResearch**)
>   _ planned assessments of IEC impact (**DemandIECImpact**)
>   _ planned client/beneficiary feedback on IEC (**DemandIECFeedback**)

Project management

31. Did the project include experimentation through a pilot component? (**PilotComponent**)
>   0: no
>   1: project included pilot component
>   2: entire project was considered a pilot/demonstration effort

32. Did the SAR identify the agency primarily responsible for donor coordination? (**DonorCoordination**)
>   0: no mention
>   1: World Bank primarily responsible
>   2: other donors or group of donors responsible (may include Bank)
>   3: borrower government primarily responsible

33. Did the project attempt to build in flexibility or learning-by-doing? (**Flexibility**)
>   0: not discussed
>   1: possible need for changes or alternatives noted
>   2: plans for periodic assessment and adaptation

34. How was the project implemented? (check all those that apply)
>   - integrated into line ministries (**ImplementLineMinistry**)
>   - through PIU/PMU (**ImplementPIU/PMU**)
>   - through an NGO or parastatal (**ImplementNGO/Parastatal**)
>   - a PCU or a steering committee established (**ImplementPCU/Committee**)

For NA: Leave Blank

35. How many different government ministries were involved in the project? (**GovtMinistries**)
      1: one
      2: two
      3: three
      4: four
      5: more than four

Objectives and Components

36. What kind of project did the SAR propose? (check all those that apply)
      1. outcome-oriented
            a. disease control (**TypeOutcomeDisease**)
            b. nutrition (**TypeOutcomeNutrition**)
            c. family planning/reproductive health (**TypeOutcomeFP**)
      2. capacity-strengthening/reform
            d. basic health service strengthening (**TypeCapacityBasic**)
            e. inputs/critical provision, e.g., pharmaceuticals (**TypeCapacityInputs**)
            f. public sector capacity strengthening (**TypeCapacityPubSector**)
            g. organizational change (decentralization, etc.) (**TypeCapacityOrgChange**)
            h. insurance plan/reimbursement system reform (**TypeCapacityIns/Reimb**)

37. How did the project attempt to develop institutions or build capacity? (check all that apply)
      _ better skills (**InstDevSkills**)
      _ more resources (**InstDevResources**)
      _ improved incentives or regulations (**InstDevIncentives**)
      _ improved information, monitoring, and evaluation (**InstDevInfoM&E**)
      _ payment schemes and insurance efficiency (**InstDevPayment**)
      _ decentralization, devolution, etc. (**InstDevDecentralization**)
      _ improved transparency, reduced corruption (**InstDevCorruption**)
      _ improved coordination within/among institutions (**InstDevCorrdination**)
      _ increased role for private sector (**InstDevPrivSector**)
      _ changes in organizational structure (**InstDevOrgStructure**)
      _ improved planning or budgeting (**InstDevPlanorBudget**)
      _ improved policy analysis (**InstDevPolicyAnal**)
      _ other (**InstDevOther**)
        specify: (**InstDevOtherField**)

38. Did the project finance NGO participation? (**NGOParticipation**)
      0: no
      1: yes

39. Did the project attempt to mobilize local community support for project goals? (**LocalCommunity**)
      0: no
      1: yes

40. If the project included system reform, did the project include an effort to build consensus? (**ConsensusBuilding**)
      0: no discussion
      1: among government entities
      2: among government entities, private sector, and civil society

For NA: Leave Blank

Distributors of World Bank Publications

Prices and credit terms vary from country to country. Consult your local distributor before placing an order.

ARGENTINA
Oficina del Libro Internacional
Av. Cordoba 1877
1120 Buenos Aires
Tel: (54 1) 815-8354
Fax: (54 1) 815-8156

AUSTRALIA, FIJI, PAPUA NEW GUINEA, SOLOMON ISLANDS, VANUATU, AND WESTERN SAMOA
D.A. Information Services
648 Whitehorse Road
Mitcham 3132
Victoria
Tel: (61) 3 9210 7777
Fax: (61) 3 9210 7788
E-mail: service@dadirect.com.au
URL: http://www.dadirect.com.au

AUSTRIA
Gerold and Co.
Weihburggasse 26
A-1011 Wien
Tel: (43 1) 512-47-31-0
Fax: (43 1) 512-47-31-29
URL: http://www.gerold.co/at.online

BANGLADESH
Micro Industries Development Assistance Society (MIDAS)
House 5, Road 16
Dhanmondi R/Area
Dhaka 1209
Tel: (880 2) 326427
Fax: (880 2) 811188

BELGIUM
Jean De Lannoy
Av. du Roi 202
1060 Brussels
Tel: (32 2) 538-5169
Fax: (32 2) 538-0841

BRAZIL
Publicações Tecnicas Internacionais Ltda.
Rua Peixoto Gomide, 209
01409 Sao Paulo, SP.
Tel: (55 11) 259-6644
Fax: (55 11) 258-6990
E-mail: postmaster@pti.uol.br
URL: http://www.uol.br

CANADA
Renouf Publishing Co. Ltd.
5369 Canotek Road
Ottawa, Ontario K1J 9J3
Tel: (613) 745-2665
Fax: (613) 745-7660
E-mail: renouf@fox.nstn.ca
URL: http://www.fox.nstn.ca/~renouf

CHINA
China Financial & Economic Publishing House
8, Da Fo Si Dong Jie
Beijing
Tel: (86 10) 6333-8257
Fax: (86 10) 6401-7365

COLOMBIA
Infoenlace Ltda.
Carrera 6 No. 51-21
Apartado Aereo 34270
Santafé de Bogotá, D.C.
Tel: (57 1) 285-2798
Fax: (57 1) 285-2798

COTE D'IVOIRE
Center d'Edition et de Diffusion Africaines (CEDA)
04 B.P. 541
Abidjan 04
Tel: (225) 24 6510/24 6511
Fax: (225) 25 0567

CYPRUS
Center for Applied Research
Cyprus College
6, Diogenes Street, Engomi
P.O. Box 2006
Nicosia
Tel: (357 2) 44-1730
Fax: (357 2) 46-2051

CZECH REPUBLIC
National Information Center
prodejna, Konviktska 5
CS – 113 57 Prague 1
Tel: (42 2) 2422-9433
Fax: (42 2) 2422-1484
URL: http://www.nis.cz/

DENMARK
SamfundsLitteratur
Rosenoerns Allé 11
DK-1970 Frederiksberg C
Tel: (45 31) 351942
Fax: (45 31) 357822

EGYPT, ARAB REPUBLIC OF
Al Ahram Distribution Agency
Al Galaa Street
Cairo
Tel: (20 2) 578-6083
Fax: (20 2) 578-6833

The Middle East Observer
41, Sherif Street
Cairo
Tel: (20 2) 393-9732
Fax: (20 2) 393-9732

FINLAND
Akateeminen Kirjakauppa
P.O. Box 128
FIN-00101 Helsinki
Tel: (358 0) 12141
Fax: (358 0) 121-4441
URL: http://www.akateeminen.com/

FRANCE
World Bank Publications
66, avenue d'Iéna
75116 Paris
Tel: (33 1) 40-69-30-56/57
Fax: (33 1) 40-69-30-68

GERMANY
UNO-Verlag
Poppelsdorfer Allee 55
53115 Bonn
Tel: (49 228) 212940
Fax: (49 228) 217492

GREECE
Papasotiriou S.A.
35, Stournara Str.
106 82 Athens
Tel: (30 1) 364-1826
Fax: (30 1) 364-8254

HAITI
Culture Diffusion
5, Rue Capois
C.P. 257
Port-au-Prince
Tel: (509 1) 3 9260

HONG KONG, MACAO
Asia 2000 Ltd.
Sales & Circulation Department
Seabird House, unit 1101-02
22-28 Wyndham Street, Central
Hong Kong
Tel: (852) 2530-1409
Fax: (852) 2526-1107
E-mail: sales@asia2000.com.hk
URL: http://www.asia2000.com.hk

INDIA
Allied Publishers Ltd.
751 Mount Road
Madras - 600 002
Tel: (91 44) 852-3938
Fax: (91 44) 852-0649

INDONESIA
Pt. Indira Limited
Jalan Borobudur 20
P.O. Box 181
Jakarta 10320
Tel: (62 21) 390-4290
Fax: (62 21) 421-4289

IRAN
Ketab Sara Co. Publishers
Khaled Eslamboli Ave.,
6th Street
Kusheh Delafrooz No. 8
P.O. Box 15745-733
Tehran
Tel: (98 21) 8717819; 8716104
Fax: (98 21) 8712479
E-mail: ketab-sara@neda.net.ir

Kowkab Publishers
P.O. Box 19575-511
Tehran
Tel: (98 21) 258-3723
Fax: (98 21) 258-3723

IRELAND
Government Supplies Agency
Oifig an tSoláthair
4-5 Harcourt Road
Dublin 2
Tel: (353 1) 661-3111
Fax: (353 1) 475-2670

ISRAEL
Yozmot Literature Ltd.
P.O. Box 56055
3 Yohanan Hasandlar Street
Tel Aviv 61560
Tel: (972 3) 5285-397
Fax: (972 3) 5285-397

R.O.Y. International
PO Box 13056
Tel Aviv 61130
Tel: (972 3) 5461423
Fax: (972 3) 5461442
E-mail: royil@netvision.net.il

Palestinian Authority/Middle East
Index Information Services
P.O.B. 19502 Jerusalem
Tel: (972 2) 6271219
Fax: (972 2) 6271634

ITALY
Licosa Commissionaria Sansoni SPA
Via Duca Di Calabria, 1/1
Casella Postale 552
50125 Firenze
Tel: (55) 645-415
Fax: (55) 641-257
E-mail: licosa@ftbcc.it
Url: http://www.ftbcc.it/licosa

JAMAICA
Ian Randle Publishers Ltd.
206 Old Hope Road
Kingston 6
Tel: 809-927-2085
Fax: 809-977-0243
E-mail: irpl@colis.com

JAPAN
Eastern Book Service
3-13 Hongo 3-chome, Bunkyo-ku
Tokyo 113
Tel: (81 3) 3818-0861
Fax: (81 3) 3818-0864
E-mail: svt-ebs@ppp.bekkoame.or.jp
URL: http://www.bekkoame.or.jp/~svt-ebs

KENYA
Africa Book Service (E.A.) Ltd.
Quaran House, Mfangano Street
P.O. Box 45245
Nairobi
Tel: (254 2) 223 641
Fax: (254 2) 330 272

KOREA, REPUBLIC OF
Daejon Trading Co. Ltd.
P.O. Box 34, Youida
706 Seoun Bldg
44-6 Youido-Dong, Yeongchengo-Ku
Seoul
Tel: (82 2) 785-1631/4
Fax: (82 2) 784-0315

MALAYSIA
University of Malaya Cooperative Bookshop, Limited
P.O. Box 1127
Jalan Pantai Baru
59700 Kuala Lumpur
Tel: (60 3) 756-5000
Fax: (60 3) 755-4424

MEXICO
INFOTEC
Av. San Fernando No. 37
Col. Toriello Guerra
14050 Mexico, D.F.
Tel: (52 5) 624-2800
Fax: (52 5) 624-2822
E-mail: infotec@rtn.net.mx
URL: http://rtn.net.mx

NEPAL
Everest Media International Services (P).Ltd.
GPO Box 5443
Kathmandu
Tel: (977 1) 472 152
Fax: (977 1) 224 431

NETHERLANDS
De Lindeboom/InOr-Publikaties
P.O. Box 202
7480 AE Haaksbergen
Tel: (31 53) 574-0004
Fax: (31 53) 572-9296
E-mail: lindeboo@worldonline.nl
URL: http://www.worldonline.nl/~lindeboo

NEW ZEALAND
EBSCO NZ Ltd.
Private Mail Bag 99914
New Market
Auckland
Tel: (64 9) 524-8119
Fax: (64 9) 524-8067

NIGERIA
University Press Limited
Three Crowns Building Jericho
Private Mail Bag 5095
Ibadan
Tel: (234 22) 41-1356
Fax: (234 22) 41-2056

NORWAY
NIC Info A/S
Book Department
P.O. Box 6125 Etterstad
N-0602 Oslo 6
Tel: (47 22) 57-3300
Fax: (47 22) 68-1901

PAKISTAN
Mirza Book Agency
65, Shahrah-e-Quaid-e-Azam
Lahore 54000
Tel: (92 42) 735 3601
Fax: (92 42) 758 5283

Oxford University Press
5 Bangalore Town
Sharae Faisal
PO Box 13033
Karachi-75350
Tel: (92 21) 446307
Fax: (92 21) 4547640
E-mail: oup@oup.khi.erum.com.pk

Pak Book Corporation
Aziz Chambers 21
Queen's Road
Lahore
Tel: (92 42) 636 3222; 636 0885
Fax: (92 42) 636 2328
E-mail: pbc@brain.net.pk

PERU
Editorial Desarrollo SA
Apartado 3824
Lima 1
Tel: (51 14) 285380
Fax: (51 14) 286628

PHILIPPINES
International Booksource Center Inc.
1127-A Antipolo St.
Barangay, Venezuela
Makati City
Tel: (63 2) 896 6501; 6505; 6507
Fax: (63 2) 896 1741

POLAND
International Publishing Service
Ul. Piekna 31/37
00-677 Warzawa
Tel: (48 2) 628-6089
Fax: (48 2) 621-7255
E-mail: books@ips@ip.atm.com.pl
URL: http://www.ipscg.waw.pl/ips/export/

PORTUGAL
Livraria Portugal
Apartado 2681
Rua Do Carmo 70-74
1200 Lisbon
Tel: (1) 347-4982
Fax: (1) 347-0264

ROMANIA
Compani De Librarii Bucuresti S.A.
Str. Lipscani no. 26, sector 3
Bucharest
Tel: (40 1) 613 9645
Fax: (40 1) 312 4000

RUSSIAN FEDERATION
Isdatelstvo <Ves Mir>
9a, Lolpachniy Pereulok
Moscow 101831
Tel: (7 095) 917 87 49
Fax: (7 095) 917 92 59

SINGAPORE, TAIWAN, MYANMAR, BRUNEI
Asahgate Publishing Asia Pacific Pte. Ltd.
41 Kallang Pudding Road #04-03
Golden Wheel Building
Singapore 349316
Tel: (65) 741-5166
Fax: (65) 742-9356
E-mail: ashgate@asianconnect.com

SLOVENIA
Gospodarski Vestnik Publishing Group
Dunajska cesta 5
1000 Ljubljana
Tel: (386 61) 133 83 47; 132 12 30
Fax: (386 61) 133 80 30
E-mail: belicd@gvestnik.si

SOUTH AFRICA, BOTSWANA
For single titles:
Oxford University Press Southern Africa
P.O. Box 1141
Cape Town 8000
Tel: (27 21) 45-7266
Fax: (27 21) 45-7265

For subscription orders:
International Subscription Service
P.O. Box 41095
Craighall
Johannesburg 2024
Tel: (27 11) 880-1448
Fax: (27 11) 880-6248
E-mail: iss@is.co.za

SPAIN
Mundi-Prensa Libros, S.A.
Castello 37
28001 Madrid
Tel: (34 1) 431-3399
Fax: (34 1) 575-3998
E-mail: libreria@mundiprensa.es
URL: http://www.mundiprensa.es/

Mundi-Prensa Barcelona
Consell de Cent, 391
08009 Barcelona
Tel: (34 3) 488-3492
Fax: (34 3) 487-7659
E-mail: barcelona@mundiprensa.es

SRI LANKA, THE MALDIVES
Lake House Bookshop
100, Sir Chittampalam Gardiner Mawatha
Colombo 2
Tel: (94 1) 32105
Fax: (94 1) 432104
E-mail: LHL@sri.lanka.net

SWEDEN
Wennergren-Williams AB
P.O. Box 1305
S-171 25 Solna
Tel: (46 8) 705-97-50
Fax: (46 8) 27-00-71
E-mail: mail@wwi.se

SWITZERLAND
Librairie Payot Service Institutionnel
Côtes-de-Montbenon 30
1002 Lausanne
Tel: (41 21) 341-3229
Fax: (41 21) 341-3235

ADECO Van Diermen EditionsTechniques
Ch. de Lacuez 41
CH1807 Blonay
Tel: (41 21) 943 2673
Fax: (41 21) 943 3605

TANZANIA
Oxford University Press
Maktaba Street
PO Box 5299
Dar es Salaam
Tel: (255 51) 29209
Fax: (255 51) 46822

THAILAND
Central Books Distribution
306 Silom Road
Bangkok 10500
Tel: (66 2) 235-5400
Fax: (66 2) 237-8321

TRINIDAD & TOBAGO, AND THE CARRIBBEAN
Systematics Studies Unit
9 Watts Street
Curepe
Trinidad, West Indies
Tel: (809) 662-5654
Fax: (809) 662-5654
E-mail: tobe@trinidad.net

UGANDA
Gustro Ltd.
PO Box 9997, Madhvani Building
Plot 16/4 Jinja Rd.
Kampala
Tel: (256 41) 254 763
Fax: (256 41) 251 468

UNITED KINGDOM
Microinfo Ltd.
P.O. Box 3
Alton, Hampshire GU34 2PG
England
Tel: (44 1420) 86848
Fax: (44 1420) 89889
E-mail: wbank@ukminfo.demon.co.uk
URL: http://www.microinfo.co.uk

VENEZUELA
Tecni-Ciencia Libros, S.A.
Centro Cuidad Comercial Tamanco
Nivel C2
Caracas
Tel: (58 2) 959 5547; 5035; 0016
Fax: (58 2) 959 5636

ZAMBIA
University Bookshop, University of Zambia
Great East Road Campus
P.O. Box 32379
Lusaka
Tel: (260 1) 252 576
Fax: (260 1) 253 952

ZIMBABWE
Longman Zimbabwe (Pte.)Ltd.
Tourle Road, Ardbennie
P.O. Box ST125
Southerton
Harare
Tel: (263 4) 6216617
Fax: (263 4) 621670